"The most striking aspect of Dee's recovery has been how far she has come from the days when she struggled to hold a two-minute NPR news clip in her memory to now completing her doctoral degree. Her singular will and determination have driven her recovery and reset our equations for what is possible after traumatic brain injury."
– **R. Richard Sanders**, *M.S.CCC, M.T.S. Senior Speech Language Pathology Clinical Specialist at Spaulding Rehabilitation Hospital in Charlestown MA.*

Blossoming Into Disability Culture Following Traumatic Brain Injury

This book tells the author's story of her ten-year journey of recovery and identity transformation from Traumatic Brain Injury (TBI). Dr. Dee is a survivor who regained the ability to articulate what many TBI survivors cannot, and this powerful account, provided in real-time, portrays the many seemingly unrelatable symptoms of brain injury and subsequent post-traumatic stress disorder (PTSD). Dr. Dee portrays how events pushed her beyond her limits and resulted in life-altering learning experiences, revealing a process of first figuring out how to live and then making meaning of her struggle.

When halfway through her PhD program, Dr. Dee was crashed into by a car traveling at 65 miles per hour. She suffered a TBI. She lost her ability to read and write. She had a severe speech impediment and significantly impaired memory. Her journey of recovery, described in the book as her trek, spans four significant periods. The road begins with the loss of most of herself. Diagnosis and evolving symptoms show her broken pathway. The author goes through a rocky road of changes in her relationships and re-identification of herself as she finds her life coach, re-learns to read and write and deals with mental health issues that felt like the end of her recovery. The final trek reveals hope and post-traumatic growth (PTG) and showcases the value of Disability Culture as a source of pride.

This story is for fellow TBI survivors, their caretakers, families and friends and professionals in the neurorehabilitation field. It brings light to the daunting changes after TBI and gives hope to all who tread on this challenging path.

Dee Phyllis Genetti, PhD, LMHC, CTS is a psychologist with clinical expertise in trauma recovery. She is a civil rights advocate for equal rights/access and human dignity for persons with disabilities, a motivational speaker, published author, producer and host of Access Abilities with Dr. Dee and Marquis, and a member of the American Psychological Association.

After Brain Injury: Survivor Stories
Series Editor: Barbara A. Wilson

This new series of books is aimed at those who have suffered a brain injury, and their families and carers. Each book focuses on a different condition, such as face blindness, amnesia and neglect, or diagnosis, such as encephalitis and locked-in syndrome, resulting from brain injury. Readers will learn about life before the brain injury, the early days of diagnosis, the effects of the brain injury, the process of rehabilitation, and life now. Alongside this personal perspective, professional commentary is also provided by a specialist in neuropsychological rehabilitation, making the books relevant for professionals working in rehabilitation such as psychologists, speech and language therapists, occupational therapists, social workers and rehabilitation doctors. They will also appeal to clinical psychology trainees and undergraduate and graduate students in neuropsychology, rehabilitation science, and related courses who value the case study approach.

With this series, we also hope to help expand awareness of brain injury and its consequences. The World Health Organization has recently acknowledged the need to raise the profile of mental health issues (with the WHO Mental Health Action Plan 2013–20) and we believe there needs to be a similar focus on psychological, neurological and behavioural issues caused by brain disorder, and a deeper understanding of the importance of rehabilitation support. Giving a voice to these survivors of brain injury is a step in the right direction.

Published titles:

Reconstructing Identity After Brain Injury
A search for hope and optimism after maxillofacial and neurosurgery
Stijn Geerinck

Belonging After Brain Injury
Relocating Dan
Katie H. Williams

For more information about this series, please visit: www.routledge.com/After-Brain-Injury-Survivor-Stories/book-series/ABI

Blossoming Into Disability Culture Following Traumatic Brain Injury
The Lotus Arising

Dee Phyllis Genetti

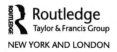
Routledge
Taylor & Francis Group

NEW YORK AND LONDON

Designed cover image: © Getty Images

First published 2024
by Routledge
605 Third Avenue, New York, NY 10158

and by Routledge
4 Park Square, Milton Park, Abingdon, Oxon, OX14 4RN

Routledge is an imprint of the Taylor & Francis Group, an informa business

© 2024 Dee Phyllis Genetti

ISBN: 978-1-032-55004-6 (hbk)
ISBN: 978-1-032-55002-2 (pbk)
ISBN: 978-1-003-42851-0 (ebk)

DOI: 10.4324/9781003428510

Typeset in Galliard
by Apex CoVantage, LLC

This book is dedicated with love and appreciation to my remarkable cousin, Hal Walsh.

It is dedicated as well to my fellow TBI survivors, their caretakers, families and friends.

My thought is that beautiful life is not always produced in ideal conditions. I liken my recovery journey to a lotus flower, rising through mud and adversity, petals opening one by one and ultimately blossoming in the sun (Genetti, 2023).

Contents

Introduction 1

Planting the Seed: Where the Rubber Meets the Road 3

  1 Setting the Context 5

TREK ONE
Budding through Non-Ideal Conditions: Off-Road: Years 1 and 2 Post-TBI: Changes in Self-Perception: Loss of My Old Self 25

  2 Potholes: Diagnosis and Evolving Symptoms 27

  3 Stepping Stones: Speech Language Therapy 36

  4 Lost in the Alleyway: Impact of Awareness 45

  5 The Broken Path: Hallmarks of Communication 55

TREK TWO
Rising through Mud and Adversity: The Rocky Road: Years 3 and 4 Post-TBI: Changes in Interpersonal Relationships: Re-identification 65

  6 Not a Throughway: Intellect, Emotionality, Control of Behavior 67

  7 Lost Trailways: Relationships and Loss of Identity 73

 8 Finding a Footpath: Rehabilitation and My Life
    Coach   88

 9 Unearthing Stepping Stones: Learning to Read
    and Write   95

10 Road to Recovery: Beginning of Self-Discovery   101

11 Road to Recovery: Beginning of Re-identification   112

12 Taking a Toll Road: Concurrent Mental Health Issues   120

13 Speed Bumps: Co-morbidity with TBI and PTSD   129

14 Ruts in the Road: Reckoning with Anger   140

15 Breakdown Lane: Impatient rehabilitation   145

TREK THREE
**Petals Opening One by One: Changing Lanes:
Years 5 and 6 Post-TBI: Changes in Philosophy
of Life: Acceptance of My New Life**   153

16 At the Cross Roads: Spiritual Crisis   155

17 Staying the Course: Transcending My Story   161

18 In the Right Lane: Moving Forward   169

TREK FOUR
**Ultimately Blossoming in the Sun: Paving a Way:
Years 7 and Beyond Post-TBI: Toward
New Growth: Hope**   175

19 Opening Passageways: Discovering Insight,
    Value and Growth   177

20 Trail Blazing onto a Steady Path: Blossoming
    into Disability Culture   187

    References   198
    Index   199

Introduction

This story is the journey of my ongoing recovery from Traumatic Brain Injury (TBI) over the span of ten years. I was halfway through my PhD program and just finished all my coursework. I was about to begin the writing of my dissertation when I was crashed into from behind in a second car crash at 65 miles per hour. I was at a standstill on the highway waiting to get from Route 93 to the onramp of Route 128 in Massachusetts. I suffered a TBI, among other serious infirmities. I lost my ability to read and write. I had a severe speech impediment. My memory was so impaired that I could only remember for about one minute.

My journey of recovery from TBI and post-traumatic stress disorder (PTSD) became my dissertation. As a trauma therapist and researcher, I instinctively kept a field journal of all my appointments (done for me for the first few years) and a process journal for how I was feeling about what was happening to me. The first few years are pretty undecipherable, but the progress of my reading and writing skills can be seen over the period of my journals. I was able to capture and collect self-observational data by writing my actual behaviors, thoughts and emotions as they happened throughout the ten-year period. This started before I could write in full sentences and without understanding initially how valuable the information would become. My dissertation became an autoethnography, a narrative story that re-enacts a tragic experience from which people find meaning. Further, through that meaning, the person is able to be okay with that experience. The story should then be shared to spark a social response, which is why I am writing my story. I was able to find posttraumatic growth and then, further, to blossom into what I now know as disability culture. It is a culture of strength and pride as opposed to the general population's belief of pity and shame.

DOI: 10.4324/9781003428510-1

My trek spans four significant periods in my ten-year follow-up. The road begins with changes in how I see myself and the loss of most of myself. Diagnosis and evolving symptoms show my broken pathway. The rocky road next portrays changes in my relationships and the beginning of reidentifying myself. This includes a truthful view of the good and bad of what happens with my closest relationships, finding my life coach, learning to read and write, as well as the portrayal of mental health issues that felt like the end of my recovery. The third trek changes lanes as I have a change in my life philosophies. This entails the crossroads of a spiritual crisis followed by the beginning acceptance of my new life. The fourth trek shows me paving a way toward new growth and hope.

I learned that TBI is the most challenging and potentially catastrophic of acquired disabilities. TBI, for the "miserable minority" which is about 20% of those who sustain a mild TBI, is a permanent, life-changing event with a devastating sequela. It challenges one's sense of meaning, sense of self and basic human integrity.

As a consequence of life changes, the TBI survivor loses access to their coping strategies. Every TBI is different, but coping losses are from their cognitive (thinking) and emotional resources, personality characteristics, interpersonal skills, spiritual resources, beliefs and philosophies. A survivor will have to learn new coping strategies. Other losses may involve: independence and freedom, the loss of knowing one's self, loss of status and loss of income potential. More specific losses may include: independent living skills, communication skills, relational breakdown and limited social support and participation. With effective rehabilitation services and integrated psychotherapy, one may again create in their life a sense of meaning and purpose, but it will never be the same. And come to realize that is okay.

Social change by grassroots organizations is slowly changing the negative connotation and stigma of TBI. Due to poor cognitive and communicative prognosis, it is difficult for survivors to speak up on their own behalf. I am blessed to be articulate again and feel a calling to share what many people do not know – my awareness as a TBI survivor looking from the inside out. My hope is that reading my story enlightens survivors, their caretakers, friends and families about the whole picture of the devastation of TBI. To be able to see the gamut of symptoms and realize they all go together under one heading – a TBI – is helpful for understanding and navigating the recovery journey forward. I also want to unveil hope for the prognosis of an unknown future.

Planting the Seed

Where the Rubber Meets the Road

1   Setting the Context

It did not seem possible that I could have so much growth in the aftermath of so much suffering following the car crash. This story portrays my recovery from a devastating and challenging life event, that of a second debilitating car crash in 2007. I suffered a Traumatic Brain Injury (TBI) and co-occurring post-traumatic stress disorder (PTSD) in addition to other injuries. The journey shows how events that pushed me beyond my sensed limits resulted in life-changing learning experiences. Unfolding was a process of first figuring out how to live, then making meaning of my struggle and ultimately understanding who I am now. My trek leads to changes in my self-perception, interpersonal relationships and philosophy of life.

The concept of growing through suffering has been a theme in philosophy all through history. There is a name for that, post-traumatic growth (PTG). PTG is a measurable occurrence of how people change in positive ways, following their struggle with extremely difficult adversities that confront the way people make sense of the world. For some, like myself, we see that, in the words of Helen Keller:

Although the world is full of suffering

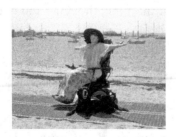

Source: Hellen Keller, 1880–1968, *Quotes by Helen Keller* | Biography online.

It is full also of the overcoming of it.

DOI: 10.4324/9781003428510-3

From my journal, I wrote:

> *I had to relearn cognitive, behavioral and interpersonal skills. I had to learn how to learn, how to heal, and to have faith again.*

I am trekking forward on my life's journey as a TBI survivor. My long-term goals have been drastically altered. I lost my old life, my old "me." My rehabilitation and home support teams, along with my fabulous doctoral committee members, have greatly encouraged me. With hard work, sheer will and their reinforcement, I am still growing in the aftermath of suffering from this traumatic event. I am building a new path for my identity. Some professionals have recommended I forget the old me, but I am trying to bridge to the lost me. I do not want to just replace it. For people with a brain injury in 2010, the belief is that cognitive abilities during rehabilitation can technically improve, but rarely fully. Cognitive abilities are the ways in which our brain thinks, remembers, grasps attention, reasons, reads, learns and solves problems. I have been stricken in all of these areas. There is a belief, too, that little to no progress in cognitive ability is made after two years. New research, though, is beginning to show that with effort, recovery can be a lifelong exercise. I am an example of a progressing effort. I am continuing to accomplish substantial gains in recovery ten years post-brain injury.

I would like to begin by telling you a bit about who I am or who I was pre-car crash. In the theory of PTG, my identity before my second car crash boosted me to make a positive life choice rather than a negative life choice. This is supposedly because, since childhood, I have found resilience in the face of trauma. The result is that I have used my own experience to help empower others. I found through my research that people who are well-adjusted before their accident will be much more likely to choose positive growth rather than stagnation. For me, at this time, though, I did not believe positivity could or would be possible.

I was a hard-working, multitasking, dynamic woman before my first car crash. I often found myself in nontraditional female roles. This included leadership positions on the cutting edge. I had to do research frequently for learning, since I was breaking new ground. I only had a high school education and one year of college for medical assistance. I had no formal training at this time. I did, however, have a deep-seated drive and curiosity that contributed to my development of research skills. I utilized these skills in all three of my careers. My three careers were in business, disability advocacy and counseling.

I also had a very strong work ethic and a thirst for knowledge. My research abilities became empowering. I also felt a burning sense of purpose since my teen years, although for what I did not yet know. I had a determination to succeed. Fueling my determination was not only my drive to emerge from my traumatic experiences as a whole person but to evolve to my fullest. This involved making meaning of most of my moments.

I initially fell into business as a woman in a man's business world. The business was that of marketing and recruiting in the fast-paced high-technology industry. I was brought up as an Irish Catholic girl who was groomed to become a wife and mother, period. I did not fit that mold. I always knew I was meant to do more. In my first job, I read, researched and absorbed every bit of information I could find in order to succeed. I faced discrimination, though, from my male coworkers due to my gender and youth. They did not welcome me to the department, believing that a "girl" could not hold her own, especially working with engineers and scientists. I proved myself worthy through my work and eventually took over the department as manager. An engineering business client of mine once quipped that I "unlawfully obtained a technical degree by picking people's brains," referring to the scientists and engineers.

I worked my way up quickly and broke many barriers. I established myself in the field of executive search and became an entrepreneur. I founded and operated two nationwide businesses. I carried out the market research and analysis for my companies. Further, I wrote the business plans and developed the ventures. One of the corporations specialized in technical and executive search and career counseling in the high technology and finance industries. The other was a new concept I created for independent consultants, which became a subsidiary corporation and national consulting association. My business lawyers alleged that I would be a multi-national conglomeration by the time I turned 30 years old.

I joined the Greater Boston Chamber of Commerce as a member and participant in the Chamber's Program of Business and Community Development. Even at that early age, I wanted to give back to help my regional community. Unlike anyone else in my family, I was exceptionally civic-minded. I performed many civic-related deeds in my high school days, including being a big sister, teaching CCD (Catholic religious class) and volunteering in an occupational therapy program in a nursing home. It is just a burning purpose within me to help lift up others with essential needs. I believe it stems from my survival mode in childhood.

I married during this time in 1977. In our household, I was the major wage earner. My husband and I made a conscious plan for me to continue my career both before and after having children. This was not typical in the 1970s. We had two beautiful boys in 1979 and 1982. I had an enormous capacity for loving, caretaking my family and to do more. That more resulted in my businesses.

I also want to let you know that a constant theme in my life has been encountering the precepts of trauma and finding survival. A liberating pattern has been finding a voice for myself and then using it to help others in the same situations. A number of the most captivating traumatic events have involved: in childhood living with substantial alcohol abuse, violence and parental divorce; as a young mother surviving a car crash that left me with paraplegia and PTSD; as a young, married adult repeat domestic violence that included a concussion, and six and a half years of imprisonment in my own home with no wheelchair access; and in adulthood a second disabling car crash that resulted in traumatic brain injury and post-traumatic stress disorder.

The First Car Crash

I was in the prime of my life with my young family and businesses when my life was suddenly upended. I had just dropped off my son from his first well-baby check-up. He had been very sickly for the first year of his life. Driving in the right-hand lane on Route 93 for a few short exits to get onto Route 128, I was on my way to my office. I barely had time to register the great big tire coming straight for my driver's side window. BANG! I was hit and spun around at 55 miles per hour. I saw the enormous tire coming for me again. The van, going 65 miles per hour, hit and spun me again. Flying across all the lanes toward the median guardrail, I pulled on the steering wheel sharply to the right. In my Datsun 280ZX 2+2 sports car, I was thrown around in all directions. I was not wearing a seatbelt (they were not mandated at that time, but that is not really an excuse). I banged from seat to console to steering wheel to door. Heading across all lanes again and seeing no land after the guardrail (there was a bridge, I later found out), I yanked hard to the right again on my steering wheel, which I was still grasping tightly with my right hand. My small car spun and spun. I was totally disoriented. I did not know if I had gone over the edge of the highway or not. I somehow slammed on the brakes, but I do not remember that. My car came to a screeching halt.

When I was finally oriented enough to see, I was in the third lane over and facing the wrong direction. I had cars speeding toward me at 60+ miles an hour. Thoughts of dying filled my head: that I would not survive this and worries about my growing, young family. Although, I did not have time to consciously think. I had seen flames and flashes of light that appeared to engulf me as I flew back and forth on the highway. These images later haunted me in flashbacks and nightmares. It wasn't until a number of years later that I discovered the flames to actually have been the fiery sun I saw from many angles as I was thrown around, whirling and spinning. A man ran over, opened my door and jumped in beside me in the driver's seat. He maneuvered my car to the breakdown lane and called for an ambulance. He voiced to me that he was a Datsun mechanic and was amazingly impressed with the way I handled the car. He called out that I should have gone off the highway or flipped over. I can't really take credit for consciously handling the car. It was basic instincts and reflexes. I had no time to think.

My whole life changed in that instant. My spinal cord was severed incompletely. I was paralyzed from the waist down. My pelvis was shifted, rotating my hip forward toward the front of me. I was now a paraplegic. I also had orthopedic and neurological infractions in my upper back, right shoulder and ulna nerve, which affected the use of my right hand and arm. Thank God I am left-handed. My suffering and loss were gigantic. I lost my body and had to mourn the loss of every bodily function, internally and externally, that I could no longer do naturally. And it had to be done one function at a time, I found. Grieving cannot be done just once for the total loss. It just doesn't work that way. It is a process, and it usually takes a long time. I became relegated to a wheelchair. After a period of hospitalization, doctor visits, therapy and stabilization, it was apparent that I would remain disabled, a label that took me several years to accept.

I became lost in an invisible world. My voice became silent. I had just a few words to express in one of my earliest poems in 1986:

Wheelchair Grievances

I say good-bye to my dignity and pride.
I say good-bye to my confidence and stride.
To dancing and jumping and skiing – good-bye,
and to all those things I'll never get to try.

(Genetti, 1992)

I had never thought about or encountered any people with disabilities. Apparently, handicapped people were not seen in the community at all in the 1980s. I found firsthand that people feared us as though we were monstrous-like others. Handicapped people were treated through a medical model. The result is that we became managed by doctors and viewed by society as invalids, no longer of any value. Perceived as sick and having something shamefully wrong with us, we were shunned. Many handicapped people were warehoused in nursing homes or institutions. Some lived in homes behind closed doors and many behind locked doors or attics. This was my new reality. Our voices were not allowed to be heard. My losses were great, including the loss of my body, my voice and my identity. I did, however, thank God that I still had my mind. I would be able to use it in the future for civil rights, counseling, advocacy and research. Losing voice, then gaining it and using it to speak for the unspoken has been a recurring premise for me. When I began to find my voice, I penned the following poem, which captures our predicament:

The Sub-Humans

I am a nobody
    but I've something to say;
there are lots of no bodies
    who need some to pave a way.

This message is simple
    and yet seems difficult to face.
I want people to know
    we're of the human race.

We often use metal
    to assist day to day,
but some people think
    we should just waste away.

They think us grotesque,
    something fearful and strange,
but we are just people;
    our looks we cannot change.

There are people who believe
    in hidden bedrooms we should remain;

away in a corner
and from life we should refrain.

These people are worried,
    their emotions are stirred,
of themselves they feel fragile
    and don't want to be disturbed.
                    (Genetti, 1992)

I could no longer run my businesses, particularly because their location
was physically inaccessible. So was my entire business world. In fact, I
had become imprisoned in my own home with no access in or out. We
lived in a split-level house with our living quarters on the top floor –
with many stairs to get out. I had never before thought about the
world being inaccessible to people with disabilities. I became reduced –
reduced from a high-status businesswoman with a keen mind to being
treated as a fear-provoking, mindless sub-human with no capabilities.
I now received pats on the head and blankets thrown on my lap, no
matter what the temperature. I was wheeled into a corner, even in my
own house. I had to make a very painful decision in 1986, which was to
shut down my offices. I have been determined by the medical board to
be in the severely disabled category, but my mind has not accepted that.
Isolated, lonely, suffering in silence, as many people with disabilities do,
became my fate. Another poem I penned, showing my confused state:

Wheelchair-bound

Here I sit where I used to stand;
    One lost soul in this great, vast land.

My head is aching, just trying to make sense;
    My head just aching, and feeling so dense.

I used to feel happy, I used to feel free;
    How desperate it feels to sit and just be.

I used to know me, know my direction;
    And now it seems I have no selection.

Oh, help me from this miserable plight;
Help me back to the track of life.
                    (Genetti, 1992)

My rollercoaster journey dipped into a devastating tragedy, then ascended to finding hope. It dove from becoming a less-than human with deep-seated suicidal ideation to the uphill battle of finding the courage to go forward. And I did not know what that would mean. I also suffered from nightmares and flashbacks of the car crash. I had hypervigilance, racing thoughts and an exaggerated startle response. I found these were symptoms of PTSD. I was affected by PTSD. My body had pronounced limited mobility, though not totally immobile. I came to understand trauma, both physical and emotional, as I was overwhelmed by the losses caused by my car crash.

From my nightmares, I began to write some of my thoughts and phrases. Coming out in poetic verses, they described my gloomy outlook on PTSD, loss and, also, suicidality. This, as I grappled with my disability. I came to find out that poetry was a form of expressive therapy. It is a therapy that bears results with trauma survivors. It was a way of finding my voice and helping me to cope and integrate my experience. The poems were viewed by an editor and, to my amazement, published into a book. My first book is entitled *They Forgot I Had Feelings Though I Could Not Feel* (Genetti, 1992). I received moving feedback from readers going through grief or loss because somebody else knew their pain. They felt a connection to me in my book and gained some relief from their own suffering. Through finding my voice, I also processed my pain. My final poem in the book reflects my emerging insight that life *is* worth living in spite of my disability. It was rewarding to know that I not only again found my voice, but I have provided liberty for others to find their voices, leading to personal healing. Here is one of my processing poems in the middle of my book:

Sadness and Grief
I Can't Handle

I'm overwhelmed
    with sadness and grief.
Why can't this period
    be more brief?

These thoughts of loss I feel
    make me want to die.
Talking is supposed to help me heal
    so that I may survive.

Life continues
   but not within me.
I feel such pain
   I just don't want to be.

I'm shattered inside
   like a jigsaw puzzle.
My mind is so frightened – I want
   only to be stuffed wuzzle.

I'll never get through this
   I've tried very hard,
but the pain just worsens
   when I let down my guard.

So, I can choose to be stuck
   with all of these feelings
and quietly dying
   instead of healing;

Or I can open my mouth
   to express this tormenting mess
and gain more pain –
   not living would cause less.
                    (Genetti, 1992)

Domestic Violence, Imprisonment and Disability Advocacy

Starting in childhood, I was indoctrinated to fiercely keep the family secrets. I had to grow up fast, becoming the caretaker of one of the households at age 11. Our family became split. Before then, I had to learn how to survive, protect my siblings and conduct a life without anyone knowing what went on behind closed doors. I was a master of defenses to hide the dysfunction and abuse inside my world from the outside world. Society was a contributor to this type of abuse by not wanting to know and turning a blind eye. I had one special spot for solace before the family break-up, pre-age 11. When it turned dark in the early evening, I would climb up into my apple tree in my yard. Branches seemed to have taken shape into a perfect cradle for my body, way up high. As I lay in this heavenly place, I stared at the stars and spoke to

God. I promised Him if I made it out of this hell, I would not treat kids or adults with this reprehensible conduct and disregard for humanity. It continued until I was on my own in my teens. I had a long list of what I would not do, which I have honored my whole life.

In my young adulthood, I suffered another traumatic situation. I unfalteringly declined to admit victimization in my marriage. Denial is my first line of defense. The tendency for trauma victims to encounter more traumas in their lives is called re-victimization. I found later in life that trauma patterns repeat and reoccur until the trauma is emotionally worked through. This became my lived experience. I again became silenced. As well, I became imprisoned in my own home for six and a half years after my car crash. There was no access in or out for me. Architectural modifications to our house were refused by my ex-husband. At this moment in time, I screamed silently to have a voice.

A positive incident did materialize while I was still struggling to accept the permanence of my physical disability in 1986. On one rare occasion, when I was *put* outside, as it was called (this involved carrying my manual wheelchair outside and then carrying me outside and putting me in it), I was put in the grass in a corner of my front yard. I had difficulty trying to propel my wheelchair, so I could not move very far. I saw a black van stopping at everyone's mailboxes and stuffing something into them. As they approached my house, they called over to me. It was a man with a female passenger who called me "handicapped," which was startling to me. I had yet to accept that I was a part of that group, even though I am medically determined severely disabled. I believed/hoped/wished my situation was temporary while I struggled in physical therapy and with at-home exercises. I could not and would not let go of my fitness, hence my status.

Larry and Carol were telling me how inaccessible the world is to handicapped people. Carol was holding a flier. As the conversation deepened, they decided to emerge from the van. Carol hopped out from the passenger side and stepped up onto my curb. Then doors parted on this side of the van and a lift appeared. The driver descended in the lift in his wheelchair. To my surprise, he was a quadriplegic, which means paralyzed from the collar bone down. And he was the driver! He was able to mobilize his power wheelchair and even ride up over my curb and onto my lawn. I couldn't even get over to my curb and definitely could not get off of it. He had slight movement in his right hand that was closed, allowing him to maneuver the tall, thin joystick on his wheelchair. I was awestruck, which very rarely ever happens to me. He instantly became my inspiration and later my mentor. I realized at that moment how much more movement I had in my body than Larry had in his. I was reminded of a saying that has always stuck with me, that there is always someone worse off than you. It helped me to put things into perspective and be thankful for the functioning I did still have.

Larry and Carol stayed for quite a while. They described to me how inaccessible the world is for people with disabilities, especially with physical barriers. They were starting a committee in order to take on this cause and champion the rights of what was termed handicapped people at that time. Their flier explained that they were looking for people to help them. I told them about my business and organizational skills. I agreed to help them with their cause because I still had a need to use my brain. They agreed to temporarily not call me handicapped but eventually were able to help me accept my disability. They reassured me we were whole and valid people, even though others treated us as though we were less than human.

I started working with Carol and Larry. Another very worthwhile cause. They came to my house often to exchange working papers and discuss ideas. This provided me with an essential link to the outside world since the domestic violence was continuing inside. I began to function again amidst the accrual of dysfunction, which many trauma survivors do. I got to use my business skills, and the work was rewarding, giving me back more of a sense of purpose. It also helped me to keep my sanity. We started up grassroots a non-profit organization designed to help people with disabilities. I joined them in civil rights advocacy and lobbying for specific issues. Our efforts included independent living issues, local access into the public domain, starting and running an accessible social center (for which we received two citations from both Governor Dukakis and George Keverian on behalf of the House of Representatives), to issues that culminated in the passage of the 1990 Americans with Disabilities Act (ADA) civil rights laws for people with disabilities.

This work was accomplished while I was still a shut-in. At times, I did get to be put out, for instance, for a meeting or to testify at the State House and for teacher conferences at my children's schools. Again, my wheelchair had to be carried out, followed by carrying me out and putting me into it. This was the humiliating way of getting me out of my own house, but it was also the only way of getting me *into* and *out of* most buildings in the public domain. Disability advocacy became a new calling for me. I spoke up to represent people with disabilities. At the same time, I tried to assist other disabled people to find and use their own voices. Even with confinement to my house, I was nominated and appointed to be on the boards of a number of disability organizations, including the beginning of the Wilmington Commission on Disabilities, the Massachusetts Coalition for Citizens with Disabilities, the Wilmington Committee for Citizens with Disabilities, AIM Headquarters and the Massachusetts Clearinghouse of Mutual Self Help Groups.

Through my community service for people with disabilities, more people in my town took notice that I was still a shut-in, even though I had been carried in and out for meetings. Several times, I was carried by the fire department, who determined certain meetings were vital for me to attend, especially as chairperson. My ability to articulate the challenges of an invisible population turned out to be tremendously effective. I interfaced with town residents, town officials, elected legislators and other advocates. Larry and Carol, who still came to my house to collaborate on projects, approached my ex-husband, who would not allow architectural modifications. They would not take no for an answer. Six and a half years after my confinement began, they had collaborated with others to put a plan in place. Funding through several agencies, for which I was pre-qualified as meeting the standards of disability, was also arranged by them. The plan was to build a wider back porch and attach a tall lift that would get me from the porch to the ground and vice versa. I had a small, narrow adult wheelchair, so the door to my kitchen did not need to be widened. A ramp was also put inside downstairs, leading to another entrance/exit to my house.

I now had access to the lower level of my house. However, it required me to go outside and down the lift, then wheel over to the door, enter through and onto the ramp going down and into the house. Their plan had taken several years to put together, especially since my back porch was so high off the ground. It was too tall to be ramped. Needed is one foot of length for the ramp to every one inch of height up to the porch. This would mean a ramp would have to wrap around my house several times, which is not practical. The front door was not able to be made accessible as inside the front door had stairs going up and down without enough room for modification. I was liberated, in one sense, to have physical access to the outside world.

I started working part-time for the Northeast Independent Living Program (NILP) one week after my house was made wheelchair accessible, which was in 1990. This is an agency run of the disabled people, by the disabled people and for the disabled people. The mission is to enable people with disabilities to live independently. One of the directors was a fellow advocate I met through Larry. John, as well as a paraplegic, was also instrumental in my emancipation from my house. He offered me the job months before I was freed. It offered me hope that my confinement would come to an end. John also helped me attain a personal care attendant to help me with personal care and housekeeping, which was tremendously beneficial for me and my family.

I provided training to adults with physical disabilities in skills and activities necessary for their daily living. Training clients to hire and train personal care attendants was imperative. I also facilitated their independence through individual and group peer counseling. I got to utilize my research skills and creativity as I helped participants obtain necessary resources, which were not always easily attainable. I educated clients in consumer legal rights and communication and instructed and assisted with the procurement of equipment, assistive devices, accessible affordable housing and transportation. I counseled participants on and set up emergency intervention and further service coordination. I also engaged in advocacy for consumer issues and equal rights.

Unfortunately, during this timeframe, my low vision deteriorated to legal blindness. My low vision specialist sent me to the Massachusetts Eye and Ear Infirmary (MEEI) for extensive testing and confirmation. I continued to have four-hour comprehensive testing and rehab appointments every few months for the next few years. Fortunately for me, NILP had services for those who were blind and sight impaired. The director of the program was very helpful in helping me navigate my new circumstances. It allowed me to be able to keep my job with reasonable accommodations recommended by the Massachusetts Eye and Ear Infirmary (MEEI), a part of the Massachusetts General Hospital. I also worked at home with the Massachusetts Commission for the Blind (MCB) on accommodations and modifications to acclimate to my vision loss.

After a period of rehabilitation and retraining with MCB to familiarize myself at home and in the community with my visual status, my advocacy efforts continued on a large scale. I became a state-certified Community Access Monitor for Massachusetts, a board member of the Merrimack Valley Coalition of Disabled Advocates, which was a political action group and was appointed to the Wilmington ADA Committee, which was a town government chapter of the National Committee for the Americans with Disabilities Act, the 1990 civil rights law for people with disabilities. My appointment was in the capacity of committee member and compliance monitor. We assessed every town building, program and service and made transitional plans for them to become compliant with the new ADA antidiscrimination and access laws. I continue to participate in these, the previously stated and other various boards, non-profit organization and town government in the capacity of chairperson, commissioner, council member and panel speaker from 1986 to the present. (I have a five-page community service resume.) I was on several speaking panels and accepted many speaking engagements. My advocacy efforts have been for social, vocational, recreational and supportive needs/rights, as well as for human dignity for people with disabilities.

In 1991, there was an unspeakable incident at my home, which involved a concussion and other injuries to me. My coworkers surmised I was in life-threatening danger, considering past incidents that I did not really want to share. They arranged an in-service meeting to be held at NILP with the Massachusetts Rehabilitation Commission (MRC) Protective Service Unit, as we were all mandated reporters of abuse of a person with a disability. They pulled me aside during the break, as I was reported as a case. MRC provided emergency and follow-up services for several years for me and my children. My ex-husband was vacated. I became a single mother raising my two boys. For protection, I will not be discussing my children further. MRC work included case management, counseling and personal protective assistance for us daily/nightly for the next two and a half very frightening years. Fear for my life silenced me again.

Eventually, my advocacy peers helped me find my voice again. MRC started a Statewide Advisory Council for Protective Services in 1993. They asked me to become a charter member, which I did. I again did something that has become a pattern in my life. I transformed my new learning that arose from my pain into service. When I regained my voice, I started speaking out to assist other battered, disabled adults to find their voices. I was asked to speak in forums and on other panels to educate those in the medical and helping professions about the signs of abuse and neglect of disabled adults. Abuse involves power and control over another person and may appear in the form of physical, psychological, verbal, financial and sexual abuse, as well as using privilege to impose authority, intimidation and isolation. Many times, I spoke anonymously due to fear. I also spoke at legislative hearings to increase awareness, gain tougher laws and protections, gain and increase funding and other necessary supports. Newspaper and television interviews (disguising my identity) occurred as a part of my service.

My Academics

My counseling responsibilities and passion increased. But my wheel-chair came under scrutiny every time I tried to advance my position. I still met with lots of discrimination in the workforce. How could a person in a wheelchair possibly hold a higher position? How could a person in a wheelchair even hold a position? How could a person in a wheelchair have an intelligent opinion? I was always reminded of the poem I penned after Larry and I sat in the mall together intentionally, in our wheelchairs where wheelchairs were never seen. People gasped and made audible sounds as they ran past us or crossed over to the other side of the mall. Mothers grabbed their children, who innocently came up to us and tried to spin our tires out of curiosity:

The Wheelman

I have two arms
And I have a face,
I cannot walk
But I can race.

I have four wheels,
Large ones on each side.
I do not run
But I can ride.

I'm made of flesh
And now metal, too.
And did you know
I am just like you!

I have a brain
And I like to read.
Wisdom and knowledge
I have, indeed.

I have a heart
But it can break.
So, listen please
And don't forsake.

I'm scared of you
As you are of me.

Creatures unknown
Are feared, you see.

What am I?
(Genetti, 1992)

I felt it was time for me to gain more formal education to establish credibility in my field. I had to *try* to rise above my disabilities. I was accepted into a program at Lesley University, which was a dual degree BS/MA program. Even at Lesley University, I had to prove how I could do my studies from the standpoint of my wheelchair and my vision loss. I was still put into apologetic mode for having a disability. I received a Bachelor of Science in Human Services and a Master of Arts in Clinical Mental Health Counseling with a Holistic Study Specialization (which meant another year of schooling and internship). I became a Licensed Mental Health Counselor (LMHC) two years later.

As a trauma therapist, with my education, continued advocacy and now counseling role, I have been looked at as a "super crip." I was considered an exception to the rule as a disabled person, for which I had to overprove myself with each change in my vocation and circumstance. I tried with everyone I met to enlighten them that people with disabilities were just that – people that happen to perform a life function in a different mode than the general population. And sometimes, we use different props/equipment to assist us with those functions.

While providing clinical expertise to clients, I also continued education part-time, where I earned an advanced graduate certificate in Trauma Studies. I kept my clinical hours always to 20 hours a week in order to have family time, along with my advocacy positions. My clinical experience while at MRC Protective Services Unit involved participating in abuse and neglect case conferences of disabled consumers in crisis. I assisted in assessment, service plan development and procuring needed resources by regions. I coordinated with assigned protective service staff in providing one-to-one support services and counseling.

My work continued in a community-based, multicultural organization that responds to the needs of survivors of family violence. As part of an interdisciplinary team, I carried out assessment and case coordination for both residential (two emergency and three transitional living long-term shelters) and community clients. For community clients, I provided short-term counseling, crisis intervention and safety planning with women in varying stages of exploring/leaving their batterers who were referred by the statewide domestic violence hotline.

In their transitional residential program, newly designed to serve battered women and their adolescent sons and siblings, I provided individual and family counseling as well as milieu support. This shelter was unique as most shelters would not take in boys twelve or older. Their low voices, which often included raised voices, were triggers of their batterers for many of the women in these shelter programs, so they were not allowed. My interventions were aimed at building strengths, coping skills and strategies, containment and stabilization. I provided support around issues of safety, parenting concerns, differences in family structures, expectations, preferences, help-seeking behaviors, worldviews and shelter daily living. In a trauma-informed and culturally competent counseling approach, I explored and supported issues related to their battering and trauma at the client's pace. I interfaced with other components to coordinate adequate medical, economic, housing and legal matters, which were substantial.

I applied for and was accepted to work on the third year of a pilot research project developed by a clinician from Harvard Medical School and McLean Hospital, conducted at a substance abuse facility. This was again half-time. I was again in a setting where there were no visible disabilities or wheelchairs. It was an integrated group treatment program called the WELL project (Women Embracing Life and Living). The women qualifying for the study were affected by trauma, mental illness and substance abuse. The term substance abuse includes alcohol abuse or addiction as well. At this time, people with mental health problems were treated in mental health facilities and not allowed to blame their troubles on or work on their substance abuse. People with substance abuse problems had to go to substance abuse treatment facilities and were not allowed to bring mental health issues, especially seen as an excuse for their substance abuse. The dual diagnoses were not treated together. They were seen as different modalities. The differing treatment facilities did not have expertise in the others' diagnostics and methods. Having a family background laden with alcoholism and a parent who not only went through the AA twelve steps but went on to help many others do the same, I really desired this opening.

I did not tell them ahead of time, the way I usually did, that I came with a wheelchair. After an awkward initial shock, I had to dazzle them with my knowledge, expertise and charisma in order to gain an offer. I had to meet with several extra people whom I was not scheduled to meet with prior to their knowledge of my wheelchair. They had to confer about whether my wheelchair and I could possibly be a viable candidate. Usually, I tried to ease into a conversation about my wheelchair by asking if they were wheelchair accessible. It gave people a hint and also leeway to politely turn me down/away. I did not want to give them that option. I again had to go into super crip mode. They offered me the position.

The group protocol was called Seeking Safety. The focus was on building skills to empower women to stay safe and to help them increase self-understanding and self-respect. It is a necessary first stage in recovery for both mental health and substance abuse treatment. The main goal of safety includes the ability to manage trauma symptoms by learning how to learn and practice healthy coping skills, to manage intrusive thoughts and negative feelings, and to cope without the use of substances by way of attaining and maintaining abstinence. As well, safety includes learning to free themselves from domestic violence or unhealthy relationships, to build healthy relationships, and to prevent self-destructive acts. For my initial groups, the project therapist would actually go into the group room ahead of me and apologetically ask if any of the group members would have difficulty working with me as I was in a wheelchair. Shocking! And demeaning! I did overcome everyone's reservations. When this research program came to a conclusion one year later, I remained at the center for addictive behavior, health and recovery.

I provided individual counseling with men and women, the majority with trauma backgrounds and co-occurring substance abuse and other mental health disorders. I was able to speak my mind and screen candidates I would work with without telling them about my wheelchair in advance. I continued to provide gender-specific group counseling, especially for those with trauma, PTSD and co-occurring substance abuse. I began to pay more attention to PTSD. It has been included in the Diagnostic and Statistical Manual for mental health disorders since 1980, but treatment modalities had yet to be standardized. Several protocols were up and coming but not rigorously evidenced-based. I was asked by several of my male clients to begin a group treatment for men with PTSD, substance abuse and mental health issues. I was surprised to have a full group of men showing up weekly for the sessions. There were several other sites for this organization. I provided group counseling for women with PTSD and co-occurring substance abuse living in a domestic violence shelter and for opiate dependent young mothers with PTSD living in a safe house.

It was at this time that I decided to go for my doctorate as I wanted to do my own evidence-based research on PTSD and the dual diagnosis to develop specific protocols. I narrowed my scope to women with PTSD from childhood and adulthood physical and sexual abuse, with co-occurring substance abuse and other mental health issues. Although I have done many purposeful matters to date, this felt like "it," the burning purpose I have always felt. This is what I am meant to do!

In 2003, I was accepted into a very difficult to get into program at Lesley University. Only seven people were accepted in this year. It was a lengthy process with lots of exclusionary elements. The program I began is a PhD in Educational Studies, with Individually Designed Specialization. This meant I designed the program following particular guidelines and with my Doctoral Committee's approval, which is very challenging and demanding. I had to write a comprehensive 35-page Doctoral Study Plan. Within the DSP, I had to select my own courses that could also be from other universities with their prior approval. Several courses were taken at Harvard and Wellesley Universities. I also had to formulate my doctoral committee. I assembled the most fabulous women, all with a required PhD. My focus was on trauma recovery from the dual diagnosis of PTSD and substance abuse, which was not an informed objective by many at this point in time. I would be adding new information to my field. I received an array of grants and scholarships. My favorite award was becoming an ELA Scholar by the Ethel Louise Armstrong Foundation for Leadership in the Disability Community for my focus on Changing the Face of Disability on the Planet. I also received a Doctoral Teaching Fellowship at Lesley University. Courses taught were Psychological Trauma and Post Trauma Therapy in the Graduate School of Arts and Social Sciences.

The Abhorrent Year of 2007

Here am I, in my living room, looking out my oversized bay window. I can see almost my entire neighborhood on one side. My flowering trees are swaying in the breeze: my magnolia, the dogwood and the holly tree. The forsythias are out now, too. As I sit here staring out the window, I am elated about my state of affairs in May of 2007. Recently, at a symposium, I presented my pilot research for my PhD entitled *Connecting Body, Mind and Spirituality: Simultaneous Recovery for Women with Trauma Histories and Substance Abuse* based on my selected therapy group. I utilized a new technological strategy I discovered to assist with my oral delivery due to my diminished eyesight. It worked out fantastically! I have just completed all my coursework. Planning to take a few weeks off, I am going to visit relatives in Atlantic City and spend a week down on Cape Cod. This will take up most of my break time. Following, I will begin the writing aspect of my dissertation. Being at a pinnacle point, I feel high on life . . . Abruptly, on June 6, 2007, everything came crashing down.

Budding through Non-Ideal Conditions: Off-Road

Years 1 and 2 Post-TBI: Changes in Self-Perception: Loss of My Old Self

2 Potholes

Diagnosis and Evolving Symptoms

Impact: The Second Car Crash

On this sunny sixth day of June 2007, the neighborhood is flourishing with the signs of new beginnings. This coincides with the next phase of my doctoral plan. I have ended phase II, which was the completion of my courses. I am now ready to begin phase III, the writing of my dissertation. As we drive by with the car windows down, the sweet smell seeps into me of early blooming roses. The roadside is sprinkled with bright tulips, daffodils and crocuses. Weeping willows are burgeoning. Spring is in full swing. On route to the Northshore mall, Jay, who is driving, asks, "What stores are we going into?" Jay is a six-foot-four-inch tall, fine-looking man. He has also been my dear friend since the tender pre-teen age of 12. He has taken the role of my driver due to my vision loss. We are continuing to chatter as Jay merges onto Route I-93 South, a road I usually ardently steer clear of.

Several exits down, we are now at a complete stop. Sitting and waiting, we are now in a long line of traffic to get onto the interchange of I-93 and Route 128N. Both wearing our seatbelts, I am nervously reminded of my earlier car crash. We just passed the site one mile behind us. That site is the reason I inherently avoid this road. Slightly turned towards Jay, I continue our conversation. Jay grumbles, "We've been sitting here for almost five minutes, and no one is going anywhere." My service dog Othello has been audaciously outstretched across the back seat. He has been lounging on my wheelchair cushion for a pillow but just now sits up. When we stop for more than two minutes, Othello usually sits up to acquire our whereabouts. This is accomplished by looking out the driver's side window. Othello is a stunning, soulful-looking, 85-pound black Labrador Retriever.

Without warning, my body is fiercely thrown forward. My head and neck sharply thrust frontward. Our vehicle is slammed up and

DOI: 10.4324/9781003428510-5

onto the car in front of us. My glasses fly off my face. My forehead smashes into the glove compartment. Still mostly in my seatbelt, I am violently pulled back. My head bashes against the headrest. The acceleration and deceleration force shakes my brain fiercely. The impact is immense. We are rammed by a truck going about 65 miles an hour. I am told later that he did not even try to brake. He did not realize the traffic was completely stopped. The sound, a loud boom . . . and then nothing – I can't hear. I am knocked unconscious for a few minutes. My whole life changes in that instant . . . again.

As I awake, I am very slumped in my seat, still being held unstably by the seatbelt. My face is just above the console. My gaze is facing the back direction. It is difficult at first to grasp what I am seeing. As I try to lift my head, I am dazed and confused, but – it is my crushed wheelchair that was in the trunk! The trunk and my wheelchair have broken through the back seat. They are compressed against the front seats. My wheelchair is crushed. My chest and shoulder are badly hurt from being yanked by the seatbelt. No airbag was on the passenger side to deploy. Jay was babbling something about Othello, "Othello's head flip-flopped from each side of my headrest – saw him in my peripheral vision – pinned against headrest now – having a seizure." As Jay looks in my direction, he asks, "Hey Dee, are you alright?"

I let out a moan. I cannot figure out what is happening. I do not remember the accident or most of anything that day. I do not remember the EMTs finally releasing my door, buckled in from the impact. Nor do I remember them taking me out and strapping me to a board, restraining my neck. I do not remember attending to Othello's seizure. I do not remember the ambulance ride to the emergency room, with Othello by my side and Jay in the front seat. I am suffering from memory loss of events occurring immediately after the head trauma. I find out that it is called anterograde amnesia, caused by brain damage. Jay is filling me in with details of the day.

I do not remember struggling with the doctor. He was concerned that my neck stay restrained until he could ascertain if I did further damage to my spinal cord. He was quite concerned with the possibility of quadriplegia. Apparently, I kept rattling on about a tremendous headache. I was also vomiting. The nurses had to keep turning me and the board I was attached to in order to target the container. No one was paying attention to my concerns. I am ultimately cleared through X-rays and a CT scan from having further spinal cord injury, which I don't remember. I am finally released, but without anyone checking my other symptoms. Extreme headache and vomiting, I find later, are signs of concussion that were not attended to. I am also told later that I was anxious and vocal about wanting to leave there after confirming no further spine injury. I passionately do not like being in a hospital. I find out a few days later through my primary care physician (PCP) that I have a sprained neck, sprained shoulder, torn rotator cuff (affirmed by MRI a bit later) and very swollen, tight muscle spasms through my neck and throat. As well, I have a horrific headache, dizziness and eye trouble with continued nausea that my PCP diagnoses as a concussion.

Home now from the hospital, I continue to fall in and out of sleep. Each time I wake, it is with confusion and little to no memory. With excruciating pain, while trying to sit up, I keep asking the same question, "Wh-ah-t ha-ah-ppened? Wwhy does ma-ah-y he-ah-d hur-rt so? Th-ah litt-ah-le tiny hai-ah-rs on the ba-ah-ck of my ne-ah-ck are scre-ea-ming when they tou-ah-ch my pillow." My temples pulsate as a relentless pounding is mounting. It feels like they will burst. Nothing alleviates each throbbing beat that echoes in my head.

Telling me again, Jay repeats, "You have a major concussion. We were in a car accident. You sprained your neck and shoulder and hurt your chest." All of my pectoral, chest and shoulder muscles, and upper and underarm, are pulled in tightly in severe spasms. It is difficult to lift or use my right arm. "You look like a chipmunk with a huge mouth full of acorns," laughs Jay profusely. My neck and face are swollen throughout, with small, tight, rounded spasms. It gives the impression I swallowed a whole jar of marbles that stuck in my neck and throat. I strain to speak out. It is difficult. I find out later that my speech is now accompanied by a stutter or an extra "ah" sound between each syllable. It becomes a prominent speech impediment.

I now lay crumpled up at home in the hospital bed that arrived yesterday. Jay is helping to pull me up. He is arranging my paralyzed legs to be straight. The bed has automatic controls that should assist in making it easier for me to get in and out. It raises my upper body and legs and feet up and down. "DDo you wwant something to eeat?" Jay asks, mimicking me while trying to make light of the circumstances. Jay is taking the reverse role of caretaker now. I feistily try to pull and slide over to my power wheelchair at the side of my bed with my one remaining useful limb – my left arm. Jay pipes in with, "You're not going anywhere. I'm going to stay with you until your father gets here. I called him. He's on his way from New Jersey." Feeling nauseous and cold, I fall back into my pattern of dropping in and out of sleep, which cycles day and night.

I haven't been able to put many thoughts together. When I can stay awake long enough to try to connect a few thoughts, I cry out in my now slowed and stuttering way of talking. "I can't remember anything. I can't think of what happened. I'm having trouble putting words together. What is happening to me? Nothing is staying in my head," is kind of what I was trying to say to Jay. It actually came out in garbled language, slowed and monotoned. I was once an eloquent speaker and had a photographic memory. There is only one thing I know now when I can recollect a thought. I feel complete horror and helplessness at having been injured so severely again in another accident – a second car crash. It, again, was not my fault. It was, again, a man driving a vehicle – a truck belonging to his employer, leaving him to feel little if any culpability. I can't come clean from the feelings of violation from both car crashes. Both times I was rammed into, and both caused such loss and pain. I am heading to see Dr. Bob, my primary care physician for more than 25 years, again.

Presently, my ability to process information is greatly compromised. My long and short-term memory problems are plaguing me. Affected is my memory for retaining old knowledge and also for preserving new knowledge. My mental clipboard is now too small to hold ideas long enough to solve the simplest of problems. I can only hold one idea or step in my brain at a time. I can no longer multitask. I must take a leave of absence from school and my counseling position. Luis Bunuel (2013) wrote in his memoirs: "You have to begin to lose your memory, if only in bits and pieces, to realize that memory is what makes our lives. Life without memory is no life at all. . . . Our memory is our coherence, our reason, our feeling, even our action. Without it we are nothing." My leave of absence began in 2007.

Structure of My Recovery Story

My story evolves through my research study of my own recovery. It spans from brain injury to the development of a new sense of self, finding new purpose and meaning in life. The journey presents four stages of experiencing the fragmentation and integration of a new self over a ten-year span. It is a journey of ongoing recovery, growth and identity transformation. The four stages and timeframes are: Years 1–2: Changes in self-perception/diagnosis, Years 3–4: Changes in relationships/re-identification, Years 5–6: Changes in philosophy/ acceptance, and Years 7 and Beyond: Towards new growth/hope. My goal was to get back to writing my dissertation as I struggled to learn to read and write again. Writing my dissertation became the stimulus and template for my journey of recovery.

The four timeframe stages also describe my levels of cognitive functioning. Developed as a guide identifying stages or levels of cognitive functioning for brain injury recovery is the Rancho Los Amigos Recovery Scale of Cognitive Functioning. The scale is utilized by doctors to determine a patient's state of consciousness, degree of brain damage and possible prognosis. It allows rehabilitation treatment experts to monitor a patient's progress. The scale progresses from Level I to Level X.

The scale is also used to develop a treatment plan for each individual, as no two brain injuries are alike. As the patient moves from one level to the next, the treatment plan changes. Each brain-injured patient goes through the stages at various speeds. The intent is that one will leave the hospital before progress is met at all levels. Recovery will be completed in outpatient therapy rehabilitation. Post-acute care cognitive rehabilitation is not covered by many medical insurance companies. The levels are guidelines, and patients go back and forth between stages. In my own circumstances, it has taken ten years and is ongoing. This is in opposition to the hasty recommendation of some insurance companies for six months. Or, as some neurologists have been heard to say, "one and done," meaning one year and your recovery is finished. Not that your recovery is complete, but the treatment is over.

I am a data point showing that people may continue to progress as long as they have the will to do so. Recovery is lifelong learning. In my research and travels, I have found that a great number of survivors also have long-term or ongoing timelines. And this is despite the negative current outlook. My recovery journey has been pieced together through researching my medical records, therapy session notes and homework, rehabilitation testing and my journals. As a researcher, I innately started writing a field and a process journal, even before I could write a sentence. The field journal documented my treatment schedule, initially filled in by others, as it was beyond my scope of awareness. The second process journal was thoughts of my feelings about what was happening to and around me.

YEARS 1 AND 2 POST-TBI: CHANGES IN SELF-PERCEPTION

LOSS OF MY "OLD SELF"

In years 1 and 2 (6/07–6/09), I gather my level on the Rancho Los Amigos Recovery Scale of Cognitive Functioning begins on Level V. Noted is that patients at this stage are:

> confused, inappropriate, and non-agitated; needing maximal assistance. The patient is understood to be confused and does not make sense in conversations, giving fragmented responses,

but may be able to follow simple directions. Stressful situations may provoke some upset, but agitation is no longer a problem. Patients may experience some frustration as elements of memory can return. Memory and selective attention are impaired, and new information is not retained. The patient follows tasks for 2–3 minutes but is easily distracted by the environment.

(Hagen et al., 1972, para 5)

Dr. Bob has been my primary care physician (PCP) for more than twenty-five years. For now and many months ahead, Dr. Bob has me seeing him every two weeks. My early diagnosis is concussion and whiplash. Dr. Bob recognizes my difficulties with memory and concentration as he tries to ask me questions. He also recognizes my confusion, disorientation and stuttering or dysarthric speech. According to Dr. Bob's medical records, of my words he writes, "I forget what I want to say, can't get my words out, can't read and retain anything." Dr. Bob also notes I am "being treated to relieve inflammation in her head, neck and throat area." The many muscle spasms still pinch off my face and cause deep pain.

It has been a short period of time, and I am now experiencing a greater range of symptoms. Nauseousness and dizziness endure. An excruciating headache persists. The sound and the vibrating feeling of the jamming of a jackhammer fills my head. An acrid taste pervades my mouth. Sleeping off and on, I awake each time with confusion. I have no idea where I am, why I am, who I am, what I am and why I have this unbearable headache. Lethargy and restlessness alternate. My hearing and vision are on sensory overload. Sounds boom loudly. Colors are brighter than normal. Lights are too bright. Vision is blurry. My depth perception is distorted, which adds to my difficulty in being a passenger on any road. According to Dr. Bob, these seemingly unrelated symptoms do go together. He further diagnoses me with post-concussion syndrome (PCS). My being is also invaded by flashbacks of the sounds and feelings from the car crash. Dr. Bob notes this is symptomatic of a traumatic stress disorder.

Dr. Bob records my simple and complex symptoms at these frequent visits. I now know that I am lucky he is familiar with PCS *and* that he knows me so well. He is more easily able to identify some of the symptoms I am struggling with, as I can't verbalize them. Many TBI survivors lack a diagnosis for up to two years or more post-event. That lack contributes to much frustration and confusion. Communication is difficult for me. Trouble remembering what I need to say and trying to get to the point of my message continue as distressing factors. A tactical recommendation from Dr. Bob is for me to write a list of what I am trying to convey. I am not able to do that on my own. Dr. Bob recaps his findings and assures me that I will be feeling better in the near future.

My referral to physical therapy by Dr. Bob is for physical therapy (PT) twice a week. PT continued on and off for the first six years of my recovery. I am being treated for a cervical sprain, right shoulder sprain, possible rotator cuff tear and post-concussion syndrome. As well, the spasms in my head, neck, shoulder and pectoral muscles are being assessed. Due to the immobility of my shoulder and neck, I now must use a power wheelchair full-time. For many years, wheeling my manual wheelchair has been my mode of fitness. It has been vital for maintaining my balance, stamina, strength and shape. Wheeling requires all of my upper body strength, utilizing my biceps, triceps, pectorals, shoulders, lats and traps. It keeps my upper and lower abdomen toned. My cardio program is doing laps around the circle I live on. I am no longer able to keep these routines.

Alas, here I sit in my easy chair in my living room. My computer is perched on the laptop tray placed across my lap. The lighting is deliberately very low to ease my discomfort with the brightness of light. The room is very quiet and still, with the exception of Othello. In his fluffy, large, oval bed, Othello lays beside me with some of his favorite toys. His stuffed animal lamb chops, one very large and the other small, are in front of him. Othello bites down on the smaller lamb chop numerous times, keeping it squeaking from its middle and each paw.

Each day, more evolving symptoms seem to bounce around in me, feeling like driving through potholes and being knocked off course. I cannot gauge what, when or how long indicators are happening. I am mostly unaware. My attention span is only for 2–3 minutes, and I don't accumulate information. From sketchy journal notes, one can see that I am having problems with cognition. As I try to write, it is in a bulleted format with only half of each thought – a bunch of fragments. Rooting out any more information is not possible. And I am unable to decipher the thoughts or fragments later. For example, on 6 18 07, I write, "shouldn't have endure severe – take away prayer," which has nothing to do with a prayer. It is the wrong word and not enough information. I have no idea what I was trying to say. I say the wrong word and can sometimes sort of describe the right word, but I do not get the word frequently – very frustrating.

Another month passes. It is now early September 2007, three months post-injury. The more I try to do, the more revealing my difficulties are. Dr. Bob observes that I am not getting better but am actually worse. His next step for my recovery is to refer me to a neurologist. My diagnosis of post-concussion syndrome, Dr. Bob confers, is also called a traumatic brain injury (TBI). Even the medical field has little information at hand and not just one word for TBI, adding to the confusion of what it is. Dr. Bob explains that my level is calculated as mild traumatic brain injury or mTBI. The word "mild" is deceiving. It does not refer to the severity of symptoms. MTBI is defined as a traumatically induced physiological disruption of brain function. It is evidenced by loss of consciousness for less than 30 minutes. The Glasgow Coma Scale (reaction to the environment) level is between 13–15. Loss of memory for events immediately before (retrograde amnesia) or after (anterograde amnesia) the accident is no greater than 24 hours. Also, any mental status alteration at the time of the accident (feeling disoriented, dazed or confused). Lastly, any focal neurological deficit which could include: weakness, loss of balance, change in vision, sensory loss, aphasia and/or dyspraxia paresis/plegia that may or may not be short-lived. The severity of this level of mTBI can cause a lifetime of disability.

Dr. N., the neurologist, is a very serious man of few words. He is very professional in his demeanor and very accurate in his choice of words. I was attempting to remember the symptoms I wanted to tell him about. When I meet the doctor, my mind goes blank. My stuttering seems to come out more pronounced. He motions for me to be quiet. He conducts the questioning. After several evaluations over the course of three appointments, Dr. N. breaks down what he calls the common disabilities resulting from a TBI at my level. He also hands me the typed report to take with me.

Dr. N records in italics my symptoms/disabilities. In regular font, Dr. N. records the issues that seem intact for me. Accordingly, my cognitive function shows I have difficulties pertaining to *attention, calculation, memory, judgment* and *reasoning,* with insight probably still intact. For sensory processing, my symptoms involve *sight, hearing,* and *taste,* while touch and smell remain intact. My communication difficulties involve *language expression* with understanding somewhat together. Further, my social functioning symptoms include difficulties with *empathy, capacity and for compassion,* whereas interpersonal social awareness and facility were slightly misaligned. According to Dr. N's record, my symptoms with mental health involve *depression, anxiety and personality changes,* while aggression, acting out, and social inappropriateness are acceptable.

Dr. N's determination is that a referral to a speech-language pathol-ogist is in order for TBI treatment.

I am missing a lot of the first two years, forgetting what I just heard or thought. I struggle to try to keep up with my colleagues and peers but totally fail. It is very difficult in light of my speech, language and cognitive deficits that tally up additional stigmatizing disability. The fast-paced world is moving on. In my now slow-paced process, I am left behind. It feels like I am always trying to catch up, even just with myself. The realization is that I am always dragging at least two or three football fields behind.

3 Stepping Stones

Speech Language Therapy

I am about to embark on my first therapy for what Dr. Bob calls my speech, language and communicative disorders. In my mind, my impassioned goal is to get back to writing my dissertation even though I am unable to write. I am disconnected from my inabilities. I am sure that I will be back to writing very soon. I am blissfully unaware that there are many stepping stones to get to where I want to go.

The office is a remote site for the hospital. It looks like a typical medical office building. Down the white corridor, I am led to a small square room with off-white walls. A desk is against the wall in this sparsely decorated room. It doesn't look like anyone's office. It is one of a number of rooms where therapy takes place. The room is bright to me and has no windows. Kathy, my speech-language therapist, moves the chair beside the desk out into the hall. This is to accommodate my wheelchair. Kathy smiles as we settle in. She is friendly and articulate. I introduce her to Othello, my service dog, who lays down beside my feet. We begin with Kathy asking me questions and trying to reel me in as I go off on tangential sidebars repeatedly.

I see Kathy twice a week for almost a year. Most of this time is a blur for me. I will use Kathy's progress records, which also help jog my memory a bit. Because my memory and retention are only minutes long, Kathy emails me a session recap of what we have done and her assessment. This is tremendously helpful. I have difficulty reading the short note all the way through and retaining it. As Kathy encourages, I have someone in my household read it to me often to hopefully let it sink in. It does not really sink in until I review them again years later. I find later that Kathy's record demonstrates diagnostics, symptoms and treatment for my TBI. She is very concise and organized, unlike my current brain function. In reviewing

DOI: 10.4324/9781003428510-6

Kathy's records years later, when I can understand, I find she has created somewhat of a portrait of the loss of myself.

After two sessions, Kathy's clinical note to me is of my diagnosis:

> diagnoses comprised of moderate cognitive linguistic deficit; mild-moderate executive function deficits due to close head injury; word finding difficulties and reading deficits due to poor sustained attention; and difficulty in speech and written language, all caused by brain injury.

One of my ideas for my treatment is attempting to collect learning tools. I especially need them to regain my conscious awareness. The problem is that I often misplace my toolbox. The tools are getting lost. I am not retaining much of anything. This includes my voluminous losses due to this TBI, which has its benefits and drawbacks. I am so unaware that it precludes any strong feelings.

On to therapy exercises. We begin our work with voice, tongue and diaphragmatic breathing exercises. This is supposed to help my newly acquired speech impediment. We also practice speech sounds. Physical stretches for voice and muscular flexibility are put in place for practice several times a day. Kathy's note explains these stretches involve "neck, shoulders, pharynx, jaw, face, lips, and tongue." I also am to say repetitive sounds into a tape recorder and listen back while I try to say the sounds and letters correctly, without the stutter. Again, several times a day.

As we move onto cognitive therapy techniques, and I continue speech especially as homework, Kathy writes:

> To review the highlights of what is most pertinent to you, here are some important points: you sustained a traumatic closed brain injury. It was probably moderate in severity [it is mild], as you lost consciousness only briefly. You were confused, and had little to no memory after the crash. Primary damage to your brain consisted of tearing and shearing of brain cell connections and probably some bruising and swelling of the tissues. These symptoms happen throughout the brain. The specific areas of impact were most likely your frontal lobe, and your reciprocal lobe.

She continues with:

> Physically, you experienced a sprain of your neck, and muscle sprain to shoulder and arm. You have had some sensory changes.

> You have headaches, and fatigue easily. Cognitively, you have difficulty with attention and concentration, memory, some language problems and some higher-level processing problems. Emotionally, you break into tears easily and feel more anxious and frustrated. You have difficulty retaining details of auditory information, which is your primary source of input due to your poor vision. We reviewed the categorization worksheet and talked about how things are all jumbled in your brain.

Kathy describes in detail the physical, sensory, cognitive and emotional symptoms I am experiencing. Upon hearing this, I am feeling confused and provoked by emotions, especially by intense sorrow. I still am unable to pay attention to or retain my holistic presentation. I am also still in denial that something big has happened to me. I think this will all go away soon. But here it is concisely, all of my many significant losses at once spelled out. As I hear it over and over, I feel like a shell of a human being. I feel like a pin cushion of holes without the pins in to plug them up. This is too difficult to absorb. I have to read and reread through my speech processor many times to try to *get* it. Tears escape my eyes and trickle down my dampened cheek as I try to comprehend the enormity of my difficulties. I feel grief for the poor woman this is written about, but I am having a difficult time connecting it to me. I feel numb.

Here I sit again in this off-white, non-descript therapy room. I am now able to sit through a full therapy session. My ability to pay attention during this appointment time is a different story. Kathy is constantly pulling me back to the task at hand. It feels to me like I am cooperating fully and attending to the session. Nevertheless, immediately upon leaving the therapy room, I cannot tell you what I just did for 45 minutes. I am relying on Kathy's notes to recreate our early work. We are now working with functional memory tasks. Starting off, I am to repeat three words in a row after Kathy speaks them. I try hard, but I can't remember any words after she finishes. We reduce the practice to repeating each word after she says it. It is a while before I can say two, and we never get to three words in a row.

Moving upward, I tackle categorization worksheets. Kathy is filling them out in our sessions. In large print, Kathy shows me a sheet of paper. On the left are six blocks, each containing a letter. Down the right-hand side is a column of pictures. I am to say which picture begins with each of the letters. Kathy says the letter and makes the sound. I have to say which picture begins with that sound. Another page Kathy has copied and turned into large print has six broad categories. There is a column on the right with pictures and the word underneath. I have to put them under the right category. One of the pictures is a cat, which has to go under the category heading of animals. Other category headings on this page are colors and automobiles. This is tough! It requires tremendous work on my part. As I fatigue, I seem to randomly assign the pictures to categories that are incorrect.

Kathy gives me the book and still makes one-page sheet copies for me. We continue in that book with other categorizing and learning styles. I have a page with the letters *sh* on the top with a picture of a sheep. There are six pictures below, and I am to circle the ones that begin with the same *sh* sound. I have pages for numerous letter sounds. I have difficulty finding all of the pictures, but I do get some. I also mistake a few. More difficult pages involve sequencing three numbers and other pages for three letters. I fail completely when a fourth number or letter is added. Another style is for me to count the *thes* on the large print page. I have about 50% accuracy. I miss some, and I also circle words close to it like the word *them*.

Kathy adds a new undertaking. She is assigning me homework so I can practice these pages. It takes me many hours, sometimes up to four hours broken into 20-minute sessions to fill in a one-page worksheet. It takes days to fill in one sheet and not always completely. I have someone write the start time and finish time when they see me zone off into the abyss. My great difficulty in finishing is due to concentration, attention, comprehension and fatigue. These worksheets, I realize years later when I look at the book, are from a preschool primer. This is shockingly insulting for an adult. I should be outraged that an adult version of these exercises is not available. But the truth is that this is my functional level. Outrage is not in my repertoire currently.

My work with Kathy during this first-year post-injury expands to incorporate some of my chaotic happenings in my everyday life. Kathy is incorporating cognitive exercises to help me with real-life simple tasks with which I am no longer proficient. It is frustrating and quite tough for me. I have a great deal of difficulty in making choices. It always becomes overwhelming. I just cannot choose. I agonizingly struggle to choose my own clothes, sort the mail, find matching colors, organize surface clutter on the table or decide which bills to pay. Even this list seems overwhelmingly long and makes my head spin. Most tasks remain undone. All are part of everyday living. I am no longer able to do them on my own. Each time that I try is new to me. I don't carry over what I just learned or failed at doing. I don't accumulate the undone failings, but the people in my environment who see the residual certainly remember and accumulate. They become frustrated with me.

For my greatest help with activities of daily living at home, I am lucky to have Jay. He is my wonderful driver turned personal care assistant who knows me very well. I did have a wonderful woman who suddenly took leave. I think she became frustrated because she could not understand me most of the time. And I am now so needy. I am needy for the first time in my life. I have always been fiercely and probably stubbornly independent. I am not able to train a new person in this condition, so Jay is stepping in. I can hardly tell Jay what I want or need. Trying to make a choice, I have no feeling either way to help with selection. Nothing discriminating stands out. If someone is with me, I have them choose. If not, I can be stuck in my head trying to make a decision for hours – and then forget what it is I am trying to do. So many times, I don't get a hold of what I want or need. Along with the other choices I named, this also happens with food. I just give up and don't eat if I am by myself. I am starting to gain some mastery of new strategies with charts, although they are also confusing to me. Most importantly, I now have assistance.

Jay is also assisting me with grocery shopping. He goes to the store and selects pre-cooked meals from the baker's section that he thinks I will like. These require just heating for several minutes in the microwave. I just have to remember to heat and then eat. But I don't. Kathy strategizes with me. She knows I have a pill reminder that beeps when I must take medication. Kathy suggests tying my pill-taking times to meal times. That way, when the pill reminder beeps, I will know it is breakfast, lunch, dinner or bedtime. As well, I should recognize it is medication time. This sounds great! Unfortunately, on my own, I am frequently oblivious to the beeping. I also have Post-It notes that adorn my kitchen cabinets with reminders to eat. And Jay arranges my lunch and dinner on the middle shelf of the refrigerator, right up front where I can't miss it. But I do. The conundrum is that I seldom open the refrigerator door. I have a Post-It note for that, too.

Back to Kathy's notes. Her progress plans indicate a few elements of my TBI that she views as most difficult for me still. One is that of stepping back and viewing a situation objectively. Another is my lack of ability to summarize. A third is my lack of self-monitoring. Kathy states how these elements affect me in my session summaries.

Accordingly, I am having severe trouble with the ability to see the main idea in a paragraph that she reads. I am also having severe trouble trying to identify a minor detail and to summarize the short paragraph. Kathy has written a strategy for me that no matter how many times I hear it, I still do not understand it. From Kathy's notes, I am:

> to relearn that shifting patterns of thoughts to solve problems by switching attention involves recognizing a problem, working out an alternative solution, and shifting the response pattern to a newly solved problem.

I also could not put that strategy into my own words or give you an example of what that means. Kathy does spell out my current goals. I am to:

> relearn self-awareness, the accurate vision of my strengths and weaknesses, and the ability to anticipate future difficulties.

I do not complete these goals for several more years after my TBI. My writing at this juncture is close to nonexistent.

As we continue in speech-language therapy, Kathy informs me that my executive function skills are lost. That statement is lost on me. If I could understand, I would know that this is devastating news. Kathy explains the utilization of executive skills in the following email:

> Think of executive skills as the conductor of an orchestra and the cognitive skills as all the sections of the orchestra. If the conductor is not working properly then each part of the orchestra may play out of order, at the wrong speed, or at the wrong volume. The executive functioning if in the same way is not working well, then all other brain functions may be coordinated incorrectly on tasks. This leads to significant problems in everyday life.

Kathy explains in her note to me that I am in need of being able to plan, organize and direct situations. As well, I need to be able to control situations. And she relays that many other executive skills are involved. Kathy constructs an example to help me understand. She notes that I have an inability to set and meet realistic goals. Further, I am unable to adjust plans at any given moment after an action plan is initiated. Kathy informs me that I blank out and freeze or become anxious if a planned moment is altered. My mind does not reset. Kathy reiterates that I need to learn to monitor my progress. She states that with an attention span of only a few minutes, it is very difficult for me to stay on any task. Kathy also reports that the functional ability to synthesize and analyze information is taken from me. Kathy maintains that I am not able to make multiple decisions. I can no longer multi-task. My judgment is askew. Kathy ends her note by communicating that these executive functions are vital for my independence at home, work, school and socializing.

I am able to maintain at least minimal function at home. I still get to live in my own home. I think I am still independent. Well, I do have people in and out of my home to help me. Of course, I have Jay. My father visits me and stays for several weeks each time. I have friends bringing meals. Deb comes every few weeks to help me sort mail and pay bills. At our sessions, Kathy is helping me with urgent household problems. They usually turn out to be miscommunications. I used to run my household like a well-oiled machine, independently. It now looks and seems to be in chronic chaos. It doesn't bother me much because I don't see the whole big picture. I am trying hard to learn to take one simple task and make a short action plan. Next, I try to follow it. The most important point everyone is trying to make, also according to Kathy, is for me to not get caught up in many incidental episodes that happen throughout my day. They all seem important to me. If I complete one whole task a day, such as heating a cooked meal, I have made a great accomplishment. And what are the other things Kathy is telling me I can't do? I am trying to find my mind and am gaining mounting frustration.

We are now approaching late in 2007. I am told astonishing news from Kathy. She tells me I am becoming aware that my losses and growing negative self-perception may be permanent. In a December 2007 summary email, Kathy tells me that she thinks I am reaching a level of acceptance of the fact that my life is changed permanently because of this brain injury. She writes:

> You do not process information like you did before, you do not juggle multiple tasks as easy, and it takes a lot more energy to accomplish tasks, hence fatigue.

Kathy further relays that it is good that I am adjusting to these differences and changing the way I approach things. She thinks I am satisfied. I FEEL NOTHING COULD BE FURTHER FROM THE TRUTH!! I am in a panic! My goal has not changed. My goal is to be able to read and write to get back to writing my dissertation. Apparently, Kathy thinks this is hopeless. We haven't even undertaken sentences yet. To my frustration, we continue with pre-primers.

In April 2008, Kathy tells me that she is not really trained in the area of cognition and writing. She tells me:

> You just have to learn all new ways to process and won't get all things back. You won't ever be like you were.

Kathy relays she considers me to have a high-functioning brain injury. Accordingly, that means I can make it in the world the way I am – as just a functioning person. Just as a barely functioning person. No more than that. She writes:

> You have to learn how to process information in a different way, and it will never be like it was.

Then she informs me:

> I don't like when you compare how you used to achieve especially relating to your photographic memory. It's gone. You have to get over it.

What!!?? No, that is what I aspire to.

It is almost one year since we began working together. Kathy is notifying me that she has taken me as far as she can. I have reached the end with her. My awareness has continued to be oblivious moment by moment, but it is becoming clearer in this moment. My goal of getting back to writing my dissertation, to me, also means getting back to my old life. I HAVE NOT let go of that. I cannot. How can this possibly be? I want more. I still think of myself as having more to learn, to relearn and to give. But Kathy states this is the best I am going to be. I do not have many feelings presently, but this harshly wounds me.

I find that the appropriate goal of care is rehabilitation in the broadest sense of the term for those suffering from a TBI. Being brought back to the condition of living a life with no parameters is the aim for TBI survivors. It is the rehabilitation or reconstruction of the mind. Somehow, retraining in order to rebuild pathways in a brain that has been damaged is called recovery. However, recovery and rehabilitation do not mean a return to the TBI survivor's pre-injury status.

Kathy emails me a final report in a session note in June 2008:

> State the main idea, predict and draw conclusions. The patient
> continues to have difficulty identifying the main idea accurately
> in paragraph length information. For sequencing a series of
> steps for common activities, the patient is improving. Sort and
> prioritize items on a 'to do' list remains a difficult area. Patient
> has difficulty making decisions about priority due to decreased
> decision-making capacity and carrying out a plan.

All activities of my daily life functioning are hindered by these essential deficiencies. Kathy tells me she thinks I have an abundant fund of knowledge, even though she states it is scrambled in my head. Kathy shares that it is enough for me to get by in the world. She admits it will be in a much smaller capacity. Just who is supposed to decide what is good enough for me? I argue that it should be me. I am minimally functioning at home. I cannot work, go to school or even have a social life right now. I am not willing to settle for this. This is not – a me, not even a good enough me. I am not grasping all that is missing, but I know I am a thin layer of the person I used to be.

I have worked really hard in therapy. I continue to cry out to Kathy that I want to learn to read and write again, that I will persist. Kathy calls to tell me that she has made a referral for me to a speech therapist she met at a conference. His name is R. Richard Sanders, MSCCC, MTS. He is a Senior Speech-Language Pathology Clinical Specialist who might be able to help me. He works in the Traumatic Brain Injury unit at the Spaulding Rehabilitation Hospital. Rick works with TBI survivors who are motivated with higher functioning and higher goals, like me. Rick has expertise working with cognition, an area for me that is gravely afflicted. I wonder if Rick can help lay out the stepping stones I need to connect to an acceptable path of recovery. The thought raises my spirits, but my awareness is still minimal. As I try to forge ahead, I am absent most of the time, living in a state of nothingness, not in the past, not in a future, only in the now – in my fog.

4 Lost in the Alleyway
Impact of Awareness

In this second year post-injury, the loss of myself as well as changes in my self-perception, my essence, are still unfolding. I progress to Level VI on the Rancho Los Amigos Recovery Scale, which is marked by:

> being confused, appropriate: needing moderate assistance. The patient's speech makes sense, and he or she is able to do simple things such as dressing, eating, and teeth brushing. Although patients know how to perform a specific activity, they need help discerning when to start and stop. They are dependent on external input for direction. Learning new things may also be difficult. The patient's memory and attention are increasing and he or she is able to attend to a task for 30 minutes.
>
> (Hagen et al., 1972, para 6)

At this time, I am still only able to attend to a task fully for 10–15 minutes. A remarkable percentage of my time is oblivious. I am aware that my body and mind are changed in a hazy way without taking full inventory. In my non-reflective state, my faith remains strong. It allows me to continue to believe that I am going to fully recover. To me, this also means I will be back to my old life, and soon. This, in reality, is complete denial. The reality of loss is difficult to face. Kubler-Ross (1997) developed five stages of grieving that are not linear. People move in and out of various stages in their own time. Her first stage is denial. Trying to shut out the magnitude of one's state of affairs is how an individual experiences this stage. It lends to the development of an incorrect but preferable reality. Although my situation shows otherwise, my first line of defense coping mechanism is also denial. I am determined to get back to – well, me.

DOI: 10.4324/9781003428510-7

I have been altered in so many ways through my physical, emotional and cognitive states. Even my womanhood has been altered and nearly vanished. I have an obvious inability to care for my own physical needs. For all of my personal activities of daily living, I need assistance. My memory and attention are carried away to a nowhere land. I was the strong, open-armed pillar of the family. In motherhood, I am now only a splinter of that pillar. Even though my children are grown, I am inefficient in caring for them. I cannot respond to them at a moment's notice as usual. I am indecisive and emotionally unavailable. My state of being has lost shape and status. When I can feel – anything – it is devastation. I am no longer sensual or sexual. I can no longer make choices. I cloak myself in oversized tee shirts paired with one of three skirts. I actually have a chart with the coordination of seven tee shirts that match all three of the skirts. I am to choose one of each. This can still take hours. And my right upper quadrant of head, neck, shoulder, arm and pectoral muscles are still bound tightly together.

My energy is all consumed with getting up, going to my therapy appointments and doing my therapy homework/practices. I can only attend for 10–15 minutes before I become incomprehensibly exhausted. I then fall into a brain fog. I am attending speech-language-cognitive therapy twice a week, physical therapy three times a week, assistive technology and psycho therapies once a week and regular doctor appointments. Some of my therapies are doubled at two in a day. Thankfully, many are in the same rehabilitation hospital.

For my other activities of daily living, I am ushered through with assistance. My memory to do or plan them is still nonexistent. My inability to maintain my thoughts and my lack of presence is causing an inactivity of service. This triggers a disbanding of many of my relationships. I am also dropped off from or have to give up on my many community service positions. Although the losses are not easy, moment-to-moment, I am unaware. Prior to the car crash, I had a full life with family, career, social life and community stations. My mind can only work on one very simple thing now for a very short time. I am below 5% of where I was pre-car crash. Each and every day, I spend the largest amount of my time just to get through it.

Much of this second year, again, is remembered through clinical notes or bare jottings that don't always make sense in my journal. I also have educational handouts to learn about the effects that are holding back my awareness. I am going to present a few pertinent *FYI* educational moments I learned during this period.

FYI: Chronic Fatigue

A sudden, uncontrollable, aroused need for sleep describes fatigue. It is an extreme form of tiredness. Both physical and mental fatigue, I am learning, changes a lifestyle drastically, especially following a TBI. Physical fatigue, though, does eventually go away. Mental fatigue is a fundamental and frequent consequence post-TBI. It causes significant exacerbations. These can be seen in cognitive exertion, chronic situational stress and sleep disturbance. As well, exacerbations show through mental health and somatic symptoms. Mental fatigue usually continues for a very long time. It is never-ending for some individuals, such as for me. Further aggravation of cognitive difficulties can happen from the recovery of physical injuries post-TBI. It can be seen as an increase in fatigue and chronic pain. Other anguish from psychological distress and fatigue display as chronic frustration, and as an individual becoming withdrawn and susceptible to anxiety or depression.

Substantial disruption to daily functioning is caused by chronic fatigue following TBI. Of note is that fatigue is not the result of ongoing exertion. It is not significantly alleviated by rest, nor can it be easily explained away. Familiar personal routines are no longer synchronized with the broader society's rhythms. Chronic fatigue usually appears with a minimum of four out of the following: impairment in memory or concentration, muscle and joint pain, non-refreshing sleep, headache, sore throat and post-exertional fatigue lasting more than 24 hours. My suffering includes five, with the exception being sore throat. I feel like I am lost in the alleyway, dark and dingy and far, far away from the yellow brick road. I feel, as many TBI survivors do, that fatigue is taking over my life.

When I can think, my thoughts are very concrete. Memory fades from one activity to the next. I no longer have world views. I used to consider that the whole world was my oyster. Now, my fragmented world is as small as an oyster. Each time I am aware of thinking, my head is throbbing as I try to force the cogs in my brain to turn.

I have chronic fatigue, and I also have insomnia. Who would even think that is possible? My mind and body crave sleep. My sleep pattern, however, is terrible. Even though I am exhausted, I cannot sleep at night. I only sleep about three or four interrupted hours a night, which is actually the early hours of the morning. And I wake up every hour. I may possibly get REM sleep during my most restful hour, which is from 5:00 a.m. to 6:00 a.m. I never struggled with insomnia pre-brain injury. My sleep pattern pre-brain injury was for about six hours consecutively.

And I never slept during the day. When fatigue hits me, or that fog rolls over me, I must rest usually for up to one and a half hours. This can happen several times in a day, especially after brain work. I have fatigue attack bouts between my therapy and medical appointments. I also have them following my reading/writing/worksheet homework and my physical therapy exercises. I have a vicious cycle of little to no refreshing sleep. I don't know if my fatigue feeds into my insomnia or if my insomnia triggers more fatigue.

According to my handouts, I find that intense fatigue problems like mine require what seems like excessive amounts of sleep. And that includes insomnia. The amount of sleep is critical for improved cognitive functioning. The definition of insomnia involves that regardless of sufficient opportunity and circumstance for sleep, the individual experiences non-restorative or disturbed sleep that elevates daytime impairment. I am further afflicted at night by flashbacks and nightmares of the accident when I do fall asleep.

FYI: Brain Fog

Another major daily problem that I had never heard of or experienced in my life is brain fog. I always valued my sharp, focused, multitasking mind which I found difficult to shut off. Here is what I am now feeling. I feel as though I am not a part of what is happening around me. My worldview is as narrow as looking through a straw. My awareness is missing. Emptiness is in my head and my eyes. I have problems understanding what people are saying to me. I cannot find words; the words do not come out right and sentences are too hard to form. My small world seems too chaotic for me. Too much movement, too much sound, I am overwhelmed. I can't see straight, and everything is so bright. I move slowly, as I do not have strength or energy. I have odd sensations in my head and odd tingling in parts of my body. It is hard to transfer out of my wheelchair because I feel so weak. I am tired, always tired, tired of being tired. This is brain fog – a mind and body shut-down. It takes hours each day before I feel alert enough to function. It takes minutes to take me back into the fog, many times a day. I am not the same. I have a great sense of loss. I feel fragile, broken. I feel damaged. When I can think, this is dreadful. I also have to be grateful that it is not worse, that I am alive. Sensory overload and fatigue take over a great part of my life.

In a journal entry on 12–27–08, I try to describe losing a large chunk of time:

*I continue often of time. spacey – zone out plane – don't know what
or 'no word.' – loss sometimes form hours – hazy thick fog roll and
cloak – dark shroud – universal complaint form.*

And sometime later:

*vacillate overwhelmedness and nothingness fog. confusion. speech
impediment and oral to writing. commun devastate. nil.*

Another entry that day after coming out of a fog and edited a bit
for more clarity by my Dad, who cannot fathom that I cannot write
a sentence:

*Sensory very acute. Bright lights my eyes inside and outside of a
piercing pain over right eye. the back of head moving all way front
slowly growing full. – have to dim or wear dark glasses – sounds
amplified – hearing all sound and conversations decibel, at same
time – confusion and agitation. booming. Can't follow multiple
person conversation – blends sheer noise.*

I definitely have visual changes. I find they are sometimes overlooked as being related to fatigue or brain fog. Dr. Bob sends me to
my ophthalmologist to get a clearer picture. Both Dr. Bob and my
ophthalmologist agree that visual problems and cognitive deficits
compound one another. Common with TBI and for me are light
sensitivity, dizziness, double vision, headaches, difficulty reading
and/or loss of peripheral visual fields, not all at the same time. It is
quite difficult to have so many different combinations of symptoms
occurring throughout my days. It is no wonder that TBI is so difficult to diagnose and to create a standard of care for treatment. It
is no wonder TBI causes such frustration. Decreased ability to perform daily living tasks is a result of these visual problems. Vertigo is
another associated common symptom that I thankfully do not have.

Awakening Revelation

It is two years post-car crash. It is almost a year since I have been
working with Rick, my second speech-language-cognitive therapist.
Rick encourages me to free-write at least one thing I do each day
and any insights I may have about it. I am also still trying to write
in a process journal about how I am thinking and feeling – what is
happening to me. These are just one or two lines long, which to

me are laborious. Much of my writing is only in half thoughts or fragments. So, too, is my speech. I am still having trouble getting a whole thought out. It comes out very slowly, exhaustingly, and then I forget what I am thinking or saying. An example from my journal on 2–6–09 reveals:

don't really – when hear a date – or more morning clarity.

I have no idea what I was trying to express. Thankfully, some phrases are more decipherable.

Zoning out and brain fog continue. But a new thought came to me today. I actually wondered what I did yesterday. Usually, my thinking is not evolved enough to wonder about much of anything. And my memory doesn't reach to an hour ago, nevermind yesterday. But I have a thought of wanting to know more, which is progress in my recovery. I wanted to know what I had been doing or thinking. An epiphany comes over me. My journal, I am thinking, is becoming messages to myself. I will read yesterday's entry and add more today to try to keep track of my thoughts. I am thinking, "Wow (!), I will be able to piece myself back together with these documented memories!"

I open to my journal on my computer on 2–22–09. I am reading an entry. I back up and read several entries and then hear this whole page. Oh, my goodness!!! I find I am writing the same thing over and over and over. I did not know that. This is frightful to me! My chest is heavy. I cannot suck in any air. Aching with sharp pains, my chest tightens. Feeling very light in the head, I also feel besieged. I have to roll away from my computer. I cannot comprehend what is happening to me. Further, I do not have the documentation of thoughts I was relying upon. I have an agonizing headache as I try to mentally process this information.

After catching my breath, a tinge of curiosity leads me to reread even more entries until I am saturated. Utterly exhausted from hearing my recurring thought, I lie right down and pass out, significantly disrupting all of my daily functions. When I awake, I am back in my familiar/ unfamiliar fog, hazy in my head and outer body, barely aware of my surroundings. I continue in my fatigue, lost in the alleyway with slow thinking, confusion, forgetfulness and haziness in thought processes.

FYI: Post Exertional Fatigue

In yet another work page, I learn that the brain uses more energy than any other organ in the body. For overexertion of themselves, most individuals have a reserve pool of energy. However, it is very different for TBI survivors. Nearly all energy is required just to perform the most basic daily functions of getting through a day. The energy reserves are effectively nonexistent almost immediately post-TBI. When a TBI survivor reaches overload in the brain, extreme fatigue sets in. I am learning and also experiencing that this causes the brain and the body to shut down. This exhaustion causes an emotional reaction, which then can exacerbate all TBI symptoms. A significant difference in an individual's recovery can come from laying down or even resting one's head, even if not sleeping. Fatigue, I am learning, is a lack of endurance. Everyday living is affected and compounded by it. If fatigue is ignored, there is a cost. It is a demand for several days of rest for restorative functioning. It is very difficult for others without this experience to fully comprehend. Overcoming extreme exhaustion in the aftermath of brain injury takes significantly longer and occurs after each period of brain exertion. So, this may happen several times a day.

With no warning, fatigue instantaneously overtakes me. I am sitting here in my wheelchair in the living room. The sun has been radiating through my bay window, warming this area where I now have a desk set up. I at once become very weary. My brain shuts down, thoughts are gone. My eyes droop, become unfocused and fight to stay open. The world is a blur. I am not comprehending what I am reading or what people are saying to me. My body is lethargic, heavy, languid. A muffled lull fills my head. All of my senses dull. My whole being craves sleep. Beyond my limits I am pushed, stretched like a bubble just before it bursts. My energy is being sucked out as though the bubble is at once drawn back in. Immediately, I am depleted, blunted, in complete shut-down. I cannot move. This happens at any given moment. More time and energy are needed to send the same information to my brain post-TBI. My brain has to work much harder even though it gives me a reduced result and greater fatigue.

In the mid-afternoon, the dark cloak befalls me – the instant fatigue. I pass out or roll into the fog. I find this is a common time for many TBI survivors, although I am afflicted several times a day. I am not aware enough to pinpoint other times. My mind work endurance, however, is slightly increased. I am now writing or staying on task with Rick and at home for 20 solid minutes. Then, I am assaulted with fatigue. I am recognizing at this time that my muscles and joints ache. I have no choice but to rest my drained and hurting mind and body. This pattern continues day after day after day. I could easily read and write for eight to ten hours or more before the brain injury. I was very disciplined with my work. If I am sick or even have a slight cold, the fatigue is amplified. I struggle to have stamina. Rick seems to know much about fatigue. He reminds me constantly that I have to pace myself. Rick tells me I am running a marathon, not a sprint.

Rick likes to point out and name symptoms and deficits that happen with me. Accordingly, being educated about these problems is essential in learning to try to manage them or, at best, how to live with them. Rick is identifying an example of my deficits with "information processing and efficiency." He is realizing when I am working past my limit, which is limiting my production in our sessions. He is imparting that he's able to see when my fatigue is setting in. He can see me slipping into my brain fog. Rick is describing that I glaze over. Apparently, I smile politely and nod my head at whoever is in front of me. Nevertheless, Rick is seeing clearly that I am not processing any information in my head. I am gently just nodding my head with my glazed look and mouthing the word yes to any question, even when it doesn't make sense. This is a brain shutdown. Rick is working with me to tempo myself. He is again telling me that the effects of fatigue can be minimized by doing work in my more energetic times of day. We are agreeing that it is usually mornings for me. We are also agreeing to schedule all my therapy sessions with him in the morning to be at my best.

Some of my basic functions that become overwhelming assaults happen when I am showering, trying to dry my hair and choosing my clothes. I succumb both physically and mentally. I need supervision and physical help. For instance, drying my hair for almost the first two years is difficult. I can't hold up my right arm due to my torn rotator cuff, associated shoulder and muscle injuries and fatigue. My arm just won't stay up. And, too, when the low force of the warm blown air from my hair dryer touches the roots of my hair, excruciating pain inflames my head. Usually, fatigue triumphs over me while my hair is still damp, and I must lie down and sleep.

Limitations and rest periods, I am finally learning, are key if I want to have energy for any accomplishments, great or small. Actually, I have not had any great accomplishments. I am still just trying to accomplish getting through the day and expanding my awareness. Small accomplishments for me are great in size. Another coping strategy is to plan and modify activities, such as censoring social involvement. I finally understand the concept now. I am learning to plan time to rest before and after a task or event. If I don't, my everyday living is affected, and my body and mind demand several days after for restorative rest. So, I essentially lose a few days when

I overexert myself – a terrible setback. Aside from my decline in efficiency, I seem to have an increase in irritability with fatigue. An excerpt from my journal on 8–23–09 reveals:

> *get tiredt trying to think – need do frustrated when finally remember – now tired to think or do – help. – threw balls for frustration.*

FYI: Filtering and Censoring

I just learned or relearned that a large allotment of the brain's energy is directed toward filtering out irrelevant information. Or maybe I never knew that because who needs to know the finite details of what our brain is doing? Usually, it is just automatic, so we don't have to think about it. Information comes in as images, sounds, smells and feelings. Without filters, all information comes crashing into the brain at the same time – a full-on assault. That is what is happening to me. The overstimulation is paralyzing. It prevents any action from happening.

With survivors of a TBI, the brain's energy is diverted to basic functioning and therefore leaves very little energy for filtering or censoring. As a result, I am finding, or really being told, that trivial thoughts may carry the same weight as important ones. This is why I am having so much difficulty in making decisions. The brain, my brain, can halt on a phrase or idea that continues to replay over and over. This unnecessarily uses up even more brain energy. This is happening to me constantly, leaving me stuck somewhere in my head with no response. And people think I am spaced out or brain damaged and unable to respond correctly. No one realizes that I am in here in my head, trying to figure things out. People get frustrated with me, and I get frustrated, too, although I cannot say why.

FYI: Relationships and Fatigue

My relationships are suffering, which is an unfortunate consequence of fatigue. My inundation with the fatigue of daily living prevents me from being able to think much about others. This is not a choice or conscious thought. I am learning this is quite common in the first few years post-TBI and for many, even longer or permanent. A small amount of brain energy is all I have for interacting with my immediate family and those closest to me. I feel more safe and at my best when I am engulfed in my quietude at home, at the times when my head is not racing. But I am just minimally functioning.

In a conversation, people seem to talk too fast, too complex, too loud, walk as they talk, gesturing, using facial expressions, all competing with the noise in the background, which sounds just as loud to me. I lose more ability to comprehend and to speak. I feel like I am drowning in words. My senses are overloaded, leaving me hurting and drained. I see much less of my family during these early years. I would like to participate in their lives. I struggle to do the best that I can. I cannot hold all that is coming into my brain to even try to process. Some family members cannot relate to what I am going through. Slowly, I spend more time with just a few relatives, the ones who know my limitations. My relationships that do hang on seem to be even better, deeper, stronger. I do not realize it at this time, but I have no reserve for toxic energy or toxic relationships. I need to have enough brain energy to stay healthy and as functional as I can possibly be.

In a process journal entry on 2–24–10, I enter an example as I observed myself depleting from fatigue:

> *Sunday: 12:30 p.m. somebody door – Othello barking – friend dropped – she takes time me to refocus what doing concentrate her – "what doing – she hugs – stopped for. hasn't seen or heard me for – she babbling – don't know what – "Noise – Noise – Noise -" turn very soft music – wah, wha, wha, wha, wha is I'm hearing – loudly. I smile and nod – in the head says "you want to come – will fun – get you of house" eyes half-mast. hardly hold heud – politely say "no you. have fun for." cannot wait leave. drop into abyss – exhausted – very muscle and joint body aches – ninety winks me and my dog.*

I am still lost in the alleyway, still off-road somewhere in this first trek of my journey.

5 The Broken Path
Hallmarks of Communication

I am still trying to bud through non-ideal conditions in order to grow and try to blossom. I find I keep rolling onto broken pathways that reveal my multitude of deficits, adding to my loss of myself. In an evaluation, I learn that with my prefrontal brain injury, I still have linguistic skills intact. Many individuals with brain damage in this area do. To me, that sounds like I am doing okay. However, I found there are many deficits in this brain-injured area that are demonstrated in numerous other ways. It is amazing to learn all these facets that are lost to me. It is even more amazing that these many functions can be itemized. My new way of being shows disorganized speech, both expressively and receptively. I have difficulty processing information. I process very slowly and then forget what I am trying to think about. I am stumped by troubles with ambiguity. I feel useless trying to learn new information. I have trouble "getting" it, or it just goes over my head. A noticeable deficit in this area of damage to the brain is difficulty in interpreting social cues. This seems to be very common, including with me. It often leads to inappropriate social interactions. This misinterpretation causes many types of trouble. Abstract concepts are totally lost to me. I, along with most TBI survivors, have lesser control of emotions. These are all part of information exchange, which is the hallmark of communication. I am totally lacking, which is why my information exchange with people is so unsuccessful. It is often met with confusion or irritability by others who cannot interpret what I am trying to communicate.

I am learning that cognitive (thinking) disabilities are the most disabling and distressing post-TBI. This is true for TBI survivors. This is also the area most troubling for family members and the general society. Standardized treatment and rehabilitation have been nonexistent. This is especially due to the complex and varied nature of brain injuries. There are many significant impairments. They affect

DOI: 10.4324/9781003428510-8

social relationships, daily living activities, active participation in the community, employment and recreation.

In my research, I found valuable information much later in my story. I am going to share it here. I found there is a complex interaction between cognition and language. This is necessary in order to be able to communicate. It is called information exchange. My pathways are broken. In order to learn and understand in the hopes of moving forward, I found from Rick's notes that it is helpful to name the processes. The processes of cognitive skills, I am learning, involve all of the following: memory, attention, problem-solving, reasoning and executive functioning. Executive functioning includes initiating, which is self-directing, self-awareness, planning, goal setting, self-evaluation, self-monitoring, flexible thinking and self-inhibiting. We engage in language skills through written, spoken and nonverbal messages. These include facial and expressive gestures. Other language skills are engaged through receiving printed, auditory and nonverbal messages. Difficulty with any aspect of cognition or expressive-receptive abilities results in a breakdown in communication. It is also called inefficient exchange of information. In my brain, many of these pathways are broken. This accounts for the lack of understandable journal entries and countless missed communication efforts.

Language and Communication

For me, I find that I cannot focus. My mind is all over the place or nowhere. I cannot even hang onto a thought long enough to realize. My frames of reference no longer make sense. Our perceptions, cognitions and feelings selectively shape and become our self-referential perspectives. They are made up of our accumulated experiences. But my thinking is gone. One of my ultimate problems is that I am disconnected. My memory is not here. I do not have the ability to be expressive. I feel like a hopeless brain in a helpless body. At this moment, I am just overcome with anguish. This is an appalling mix with my other TBI and PTSD symptoms. Some individuals find strength from traumatic and adverse experiences. Not for me at this point in time. I wonder in my journal:

> *How do I reconnect the wood [world] so many [disconnections] and missing memories?*
>> (I filled in two right and missing words.)

Communication is our link to the outside world. And now it seems mine is severed. Since after the car crash, I have had a tough time communicating my needs to the people in my life. I am affected in speaking, reading, gesturing and writing. My inability to process language interferes with both written and spoken language. I am having difficulty understanding passages of text that are simple to read pre-TBI. This comprises my own research and writing. I recognize the work as well written but do not understand the content. I do not recognize it as mine. It is overwhelming. My communicative skills have become diminutive – pocket-sized.

Through Rick's progress notes at this time, I am alerted that I have ineffective problem-solving abilities. He also notes disorganization in my head. Contributing to my interference, Rick adds inflexibility and impulsivity. Rick uncovered other common obstructions for TBI survivors that are affecting me. They include inadequate retrieval of stored or old information and difficulty processing abstract information.

I am suffering the greatest losses and, ultimately, the most negative changes in my self-perception. It is visible, according to my speech therapist, through my losses in the five cognitive domain areas. I have lost myself and cannot get back to me. Each day, I swiftly feel more of me slipping away until I hardly know myself. I no longer have my memories. Fewer journal entries are comprehendible. I am grateful that Rick has kept my speech therapy sessions and homework. I am very debilitated, causing poor quality of life and increased dependency. I have a failure to function at a higher level. I have always strived to function at the highest level. I am putting this story together by researching all of my medical records, therapy session notes and written homework.

Miscommunication

Miscommunication happens all the time now. Trying to remember what I want to say with my diminutive mental clipboard is irritating. Leaving out important pieces of information, the details, I am difficult to understand. I speak and write in half thoughts. It is still difficult for me to find the words I want to say. I get a hold of a thought in my head. I can only drag out a small part of it to say, and very slowly. My speech is so slow that people think I have finished my thought way before I do. Even when it does not make sense, they accept it as the "new normal" for me. I am accepted or ignored as senseless. I am dismissed. Or they cut me off and inaccurately finish my sentence. Another struggle is, on the one hand, snatching a fragment of the racing and flooding thoughts I sometimes have. On the other hand, I am trying to relay the emptiness in my brain, which is a complete blank slate. The racing, flooding thoughts, to me, can be likened to very loud noise, akin to turning the channels of the radio fast with the volume way up and not settling on a station. Nor are they even able to be heard enough to understand what is being said or sung – just earsplitting static. Sometimes, I even know what I want to say in my head, but it is too exhausting to get it out. I am imprisoned with half-thoughts. I am dreadfully fatigued. It is easier, less exhausting and less frustrating to not even try to speak. Therefore, my silence and isolation continue.

According to my journal hen-scratching, hearing two people talk at the same time is very loud. It causes me confusion. I cannot tell what either or both are saying. It hurts my head. It causes a huge headache in my frontal lobe. I have a hard time making out what any new information or new learning is. I can only tolerate small stimulation. When two people are talking, it is received by me like people talking a foreign language *at* me. Oh, but I yearn for the old, astute, well-spoken, reflective, intelligent brain/person. I have literally lost my mind.

My miscommunication happens with my doctors, as well. I cannot think fast enough to answer their questions within the time constraint of an appointment. And I do not remember what I want to discuss. Not enough words come out to make sense. Pouring my thoughts out and information processing is analogous to pouring water through a funnel. Information coming in through the top goes out slower through the narrowed bottom. It eventually overflows if I keep filling the top. The result is overflowing, garbled language. I try to write notes to bring, but I physically have difficulty putting the pen and words to the paper. I try to tell my PCP that "I'm still in here, me, not this new me." I only manage to draw tears. This is very unlike my pre-injury self. I feel as though I am a foreigner in my own country/world/culture. Every form of communication is too difficult. Confusion, miscommunication, frustration.

I tried to communicate the idea of writing a note for my doctor in my journal. It was on 5–28–09, almost two years to the date of my accident. My free-style sentence is longer. However, clarity is still missing. How will I ever get back to writing my dissertation? Journal entry:

> *I couldn't I realize couldn't write so thought everything involved so practiced – physically and so someone said write down didn't know wh but also then though of but too had to leave room if I got _____ (?) so said and yes – overwhelmed.*

According to Rick's progress notes in 2008, social communication is very difficult for me. Rick recorded that maintaining a topic, interpreting subtleties of the conversation, taking turns speaking, keeping up with others at a seemingly rapid rate of conversation and using a suitable tone of voice are areas for me to work on. I have to first break down longer messages into smaller pieces. Understanding one whole sentence is too much information for my memory capacity just now. Rick is teaching me to break sentences down into three parts. They are usually the subject, verb and object. I am then to repeat or rehearse messages to ensure I have processed all the critical information. That is crucial but complicated for me. Other targeted functions we are to work on involve auditory comprehension and verbal expression.

An example of my social miscommunication happens. I am sitting at my kitchen table with two of my Lesley University cohorts. We are trying to have a conversation. Shame fills my insides as I try to interact with them. I am not as capable as before my car crash. A barrage of words comes speeding at me as a voluminous attack. It feels like they are choking me. There is too much talking around me or at me. I cannot always respond. When I finally comprehend, I am too slow at gathering my thoughts and getting my words out of my mouth. My friends are onto a different subject. I am misunderstanding what is being said. When I reply, it seems totally off base. People who do not know me view me as either mentally slow or mentally retarded. Miscommunication happens every day. It is easier to just not talk.

FYI: Memory

In this timeframe, most of my journal entries are still undecipherable. According to Rick's notes, though, I had to learn about memory function in order to improve it. I hope I am not boring in this chapter. Much of this chapter is about what I had to learn in order to communicate in a way in which people would understand me. I felt in my head that people should understand me, but this rote learning helped teach me what I had to do to expand my communication and understanding skills. Rick taught me there are a number of processes that interfere with memory disorders, affecting cognitive and communicative abilities. They include new learning, relearning, recall and rote memory. So, I try with great effort to hold information in my head. Manipulation of thoughts, though, is either very time-consuming, or I forget them. For example, when I try to hold more than one idea, I quickly use up my brain capacity. My new task, according to Rick is first to fully understand and remember one idea.

Next, after I "get that," I take notes to consolidate my new knowledge or "renewed knowledge." Then, I have to work on the next idea. If they are similar, I can now, many times, assimilate them after much practice and trials of memorization. This is tedious.

Trying to integrate cognitive as well as emotional ideas is actually painful. I get a pounding headache in my temples. I squint. My eyes strain as they feel like they cross. It seems like I am trying to will parts of my brain to cooperate with the others. It is difficult to make that cross-over. I see these different ideas almost as enemies that will not cooperate with each other. I try a litany of external memory aids. They are compensatory strategies such as: a memory notebook, memory log, to-do lists, calendar, feelings log, transportation numbers and names. I also try assistive technology tools such as: voice recorders, my personal computer and other portable electronic devices.

FYI: Attention

From Rick, I am learning that attention is the foundation of memory function. In Rick's progress notes in 2008, I find it is more difficult for me to focus on simple tasks. It is difficult for me to remember to perform my daily routines on a given day in a manner that is efficient and effective. This is apparently due to trouble paying attention. According to Rick, self-monitoring is an important factor in recovery. My capability is compromised, making it harder to monitor my thoughts and behaviors. Retraining my brain to improve functioning will involve exercising the overlap of attention, memory and executive functions.

It seemed to me that the effort of paying attention was just one step. But from Rick, I am learning that there are six different types of attention. Concentration, which is *sustained* or *focused attention*, is the application of a mental effort in a sustained, purposeful manner. This is used, for example, when I am listening to a book for reading. The ability to perform two different tasks simultaneously is called *divided attention*. This is used when listening to more than one person talking. Detecting rarely occurring signals over a prolonged period of time is called *vigilant attention*. It is that ability that is utilized, such as when I am watching shooting stars. The ability to switch from one stimulus to another is called *alternating* or *switching attention*. An example of its use is when I am finishing reading a chapter in my book while keeping an eye on the time. *Selective attention* is the ability to listen to one stimulus, such as a book, while completely blocking out another, such as a crowded waiting room.

Attention is complex. It is something most people never have to define or dissect. With deficits in all of these types of attention, all of these broken paths, it is much clearer to understand what and why I don't understand. Learning about the types of attention gives me insight to hopefully become more capable of expanding my capacity. I feel like the retraining exercises of my brain are improving my attention more as time goes by. I am laboring to connect myself back to the main road or to at least find a beaten pathway.

I took simple, everyday tasks for granted until my brain became damaged. I now try to concentrate on thinking through a single task or thought in my head. At times, I try to write it down so I can look for the possibilities involved. I still lose focus easily. This makes everyday tasks extraordinary. For instance, when I try to make a phone appointment, it is now a two-day or more multitask undertaking. To speak, comprehend, think and process visual input is very difficult – complicated. I never used the word *difficult* in my vocabulary pre-TBI. I was up for every challenge – always. So now, I look at my calendar to determine which days I can potentially go to the appointment. I write it down. I then determine who can take me as I cannot drive. I have to find out their availability and write that down in the same place (sometimes, I scatter my notes on several pieces of paper and then lose them). Next, I write down what I need to ask the doctor's office and their phone number. This is exhausting and overwhelming, leaving me totally fatigued. I am now literally unable to place the phone call. This has been a momentous effort. I must rest. This is my new life.

I try to make the call the next day. Most often, I am unsuccessful in my follow-up due to non-decipherable bullet-point notes. At the time, I thought I was very clear. After repeating the note-taking process, I make the phone call. If the office gives me an alternate date from my available times, I cannot think through the alternatives while on the phone. I write down their alternate dates and times and have to call them back. My writing is labored and slow. I hang up and try to reprocess their alternatives. Exhausted from hearing the changes, I then have to check with my driver's times and then eventually look at my calendar again. I have to call the doctor's office back. It usually has to be another day, though, as I am totally fatigued again. Along the way, the appointment gets made, or I have someone else do it for me as my stamina is depleted.

FYI: Sensory Function and Communication

More learning. This particular chapter is full of new learning that I gleaned from my records, as my journal entries at this point are still not decipherable. As I learn the nitty-gritty about communication, it becomes easier for me to write my thoughts in a more cohesive way, even though still in bullet points. Did you know that the senses are the first step in thinking? It is labeled visual scanning. This allows us to process and monitor the data in the environment surrounding us. For me, the ability to perform simple skill-oriented tasks is affected by my altered and damaged sensory perception. As well, my ability to perform complex intellectual responsibilities is deeply affected.

I am finding there are many sensitivities that challenge an individual with a brain injury. An instance can happen while shopping or dining out. The brain may shut down due to background music, fluorescent lights and much more visual stimuli. The most important solution seems to be getting to a quiet place and resting one's brain after the experience. There is a hypersensitivity to sound that causes the auditory system to be very sensitive to environmental noise. Going to social gatherings, restaurants and even the grocery store, I find, are great causes for difficulty. Many TBI survivors stay at home or go out to places that are less crowded and less noisy. This helps to avoid the assault and feeling overwhelmed. Another cause of the feeling of assault or being overwhelmed are common noises at home. Such noises can be from a heating system, vibrating refrigerator, humming fan or even the air conditioner. I am learning that planning social activities when there are fewer people around and less commotion makes for a more successful outing for a TBI survivor.

A case in point: I am in a Best Buy store. Everything sounds so terribly loud, and at once, I hear: multiple people's conversations from all around the store, the ceiling fans, the metal sound of people touching the washers and dryers, people taking steps walking on the floor, the salesperson's pitch. All the lights are far too bright. It is an assault. It is too much, too overloading, too overstimulating. I am overwhelmed and overcome. Everything is spinning. I have to immediately leave the store before I can even comprehend what is happening. Another second occasion happens in Rick's office. I hear the quiet baseboard heat very loudly, Rick clicking the mouse on his computer, the different clicks of the keys on his keyboard loudly, the clock ticking, which no one else hears. I also hear the ring of the phone and Meredith, Rick's speech therapy intern, talking, all at once and equally as loud, amplified. It becomes consuming and insufferable. Rick modifies the environment to lessen the impact. He pulls down the shade, dims the light and shuts the door.

FYI: Motor Function and Communication

More effects on communication. I am learning that residual motor impairments affect the act of handwriting tasks. I have even more broken paths. These paths impact a TBI survivor's ability to reacquire writing skills and accomplish written language. I am finding that my computer keyboard is challenging. It is cognitively demanding and fatiguing. I have to devote major resources to the motor functioning of typing. Therefore, the amount of remaining cognitive resources to generate content is limited.

One cognitive deficit can substantially affect the quality of written language and writing tasks. My many cognitive deficits include my language processing difficulties. I am struggling to write or speak what I am trying to think and convey. I can't stress how extremely frustrating and debilitating this is. Speech-generating devices (SGD) are recommended over other writing systems. They help limit the frequency of shifting between the creative and the technical aspects of writing. Smaller quantities of text are usually produced but with greater ease. My memory impairments, however, negatively affect my ability to functionally use a speech recognition processor. I work effortfully with my assistive technology therapist, Rachael. I have days of "getting it" and then "losing it" with Dragon Naturally Speaking. Our working goals are to regain my thoughts, be able to hold onto words long enough to say a whole thought, and capture ideas. I am improving in fluency, note taking, my memory and technology capabilities. I have to take voluminous breaks and need much perseverance. This is all exceptionally demanding. It is also the basics for me to try to get back to me. Or for me to have any productivity.

The Final FYI: Perceived Assumptions and Attitudes

Looking through the lens of PTG, I find that many trauma survivors describe a change in the way they envision themselves. It is described through strength, wisdom and a greater sense of resiliency. They also report a greater acceptance of their limitations and vulnerabilities. At this stage, I do not realize any of these. I don't have a clear vision of who I am anymore. I am still not fully aware of many of my symptoms and disabilities, nor of any positivity. I am not aware of the whole picture. I am very numb and very forgetful from one minute to the next.

I still, however, hang onto my irrational thoughts that I will be back to writing my dissertation. This, I am assuming, will get me my old life back and in the very near future. I am mortified in one minute at my lack of – and slow – progress. I am then calm and vague in the next moment in my nothingness fog. Information is not carrying over. I just do not know – much of anything. I have no conscious perception of myself as a human being. I am starting to add up some of the losses, most of which is the loss of my "old self." I do know that I do not accept this as a permanent me. I miss myself dearly. With this, I have no coping skills, no growth or rebuilding, and no strength or wisdom from my trauma in these first two years. My resilience is but a shadow. It happened, and here I am. I keep working on my therapies. My strength and confidence are but a flicker. My denial is a flame.

A self-evaluative journal entry towards the end of this second year:

> *Try my head fix – all physical pain down to one limb – who carry this way? Exhaustion continues its hide from you do anything and I probably should call the doctor – have no energy . . . feel concave – just lumped – my body just turning inward – and down.*

And later that day:

> *This hard to admit – I feel very stupid – try is to its very insignificant, a failure, a disappointment – I weary – crushed my spirit.*

My assumptive world is shattered. I no longer believe the world is predictable or safe. Life is meaningless. Events do not make sense to me. It seems that I have no control over my life. Viewing people as basically kindhearted no longer resonates as true. The random acts of violence in my life have recurred by men who are not affected by their actions. I feel that I was a good, moral, capable and worthy person. So why did this happen? How do I rebuild my sensory and perspective worldviews? Or do I? Becoming more self-aware in early 2009, I still suffer tremendously from the loss of what seems like most of me. I perceive no growth. Depressive and overwhelming feelings are growing. I am told it is possible to keep working on strategies to have a productive life, albeit with difficulty. I am beginning to wonder if I have to develop a new self or wallow in self-pity. I am not a wallower. Needing more reconstruction are my shattered assumptions of the world. Often following that, consequently, are changes in self-perception. This did not occur for me in these first two years.

Trek Two

Rising through Mud and Adversity: The Rocky Road

Years 3 and 4 Post-TBI: Changes in Interpersonal Relationships: Re-identification

6 Not a Throughway
Intellect, Emotionality, Control of Behavior

In years 3 and 4 (end/2009, 2010, 2011), I progress to Level VII on the Rancho Los Amigos Recovery Scale (RLAS) marked as:

> automatic appropriate, needing minimal assistance for daily living skills. The patient can perform all self-care activities and are usually coherent. They have difficulty remembering recent events and discussions. If physically able, patients can carry out routine activities. Rational judgments, calculations, and solving multi-step problems present difficulties, yet patients may not seem to realize this. They need supervision for safety.
>
> (Hagen et al., 1972, para 7)

I still need assistance with activities of daily living due to continued injuries in my head-neck-shoulder-pectoral muscle groups. The injuries preclude me from raising and moving my arm up or out to the side or toward my back, using my bicep and hand and putting pressure on my arm for lifting myself to transfer in and out of my wheelchair. I still need assistance with transfers. I have my second rotator cuff surgery in December 2009, which causes a lot of physical debilitations, as I am left with just one good working limb, my left arm. Recovery is prolonged and not greatly successful. The rest of the above description for this level on the RLAS for this third and fourth year are precise.

In the culture of TBI and PTSD, there are many overlapping symptoms. A few of my pervasive symptoms in this time frame include: memory troubles, word findings, distractibility, fatigue, problem-solving difficulties, photophobia, interpersonal

DOI: 10.4324/9781003428510-10

difficulties, depression, anxiety, insomnia, irritability/anger, trouble concentrating, hyperarousal and avoidance. Communication continues to be an acute problem. I have a continued speech impediment. I also repeat myself unknowingly or become verbose. Trying to understand written as well as spoken messages is an arduous struggle. I have more difficulty with reading, writing and spelling. To use these previously second-nature communication skills is comparable to learning a new language. I am learning that I, as well as other TBI survivors, am silenced both in lack of communication skills and a lack of medical knowledge, treatment and research in order for me to heal. Moreover, the embarrassment of feeling like a different person and the stigma associated with both TBI and PTSD adds to the accounts for my silence. My isolation expands. In this time span, I do things over and over and over, but each time is new to me. I learn and I forget strategies to help me remember. I am going down pathways but finding no throughways.

In these third and fourth years post-TBI, I am given a Brain Injury Checklist, a self-assessment of neuropsychological impairments caused by brain injuries that can increase self-awareness. It can be used to track and measure TBI impairments problematic to me and also improvement over time. I cannot, in this time frame, keep up with the checklist form daily or even weekly. I have to think too long for each item to try to recall what I experience each day, then make a selection on a severity score. This simple type of brain work is beyond my brain capacity at this time. It takes an inordinate amount of time. I cannot recall and cannot make a decision/judgment/selection. Further, notes can be made for what makes the impairments worse or better. The checklist is a tool to increase awareness and to assist in memory and restoring intellectual skills. It is highly frustrating and anxiety-provoking as I try to do these tasks. Therefore, I do not. However, I can see that I have an overwhelming number of impairments, but it does not register with me consciously. In retrospect, I experienced a greater amount of the more troublesome ones on some days, making me totally dysfunctional and less symptomatic on others, wherein I can be higher functioning, which is typical post-TBI.

I learn from the checklist, three more years in the future, that there are three functional systems that characterize neurological impairments caused by brain injury. They are: (1) intellect – the information-handling facet of behavior; (2) emotionality – pertaining to feelings and motivations; and (3) control – how behavior is expressed. Regardless of the size or location of the TBI, brain damage usually affects all three systems. There are six groups of persistent suffering/ impairments, inclusive of neuropsychological problems affecting intellect. It is helpful to name them: persistent intellectual impairments, psychological consequences, persistent mood disorders, persistent physiological impairments, persistent personality alterations and persistent neurological problems. My daily life consists of many of these impairments.

Some of the consequences in my daily functioning, including the next few instances, are illustrative of persistent intellectual impairments. My files are as disorganized as my brain. Forever misplacing my effects, I have enormous difficulty tracking them. Extremely exacerbating, I have tried abundant strategies. With the exception of the stratagem of writing things down, I do not remember most of these third and fourth years. Added troubles occur when I try to remember what I want to write and where I put the note, even on my computer. Too often, I cannot remember or even guess what I named a file. Nor can I remember what category I filed it under in my computer and file drawer. Tracking what I need for a grocery list is futile. I, too, am forever misplacing bills, the mail, phone messages, the phone, writing drafts and household equipment. Pre-TBI, I was extremely organized, especially due to my sight. I also had a photographic memory that I took for granted. After a series of failed attempts, I now work with Rick for retraining in each area.

Surveying my difficulty in making decisions demonstrates that I produce either very late or no responses due in part to slow processing. Many times, I just cannot make choices. The values are the same. Nothing stands out. I cannot prioritize. I cannot justify whether to pay a bill right now or go try to pick out a shirt to wear, as they have the same import to me. They all take an inordinate amount of time. Now and then when I am asked a choice, my mind goes completely blank, and at times, I just hear, "Do you want 'static' or 'static.'"

Finally, I become disoriented by slight changes in my daily routine. When I have in mind a fixed order of doing something, it is challenging and flustering to switch gears. Trying to process a change of information takes me a long time in order to readjust to a new thought or scenario. It is like slow, rusty gears churning in my brain to line up with the new information. This can cause confusion and agitation. I become unsure about things that I know well. From the brain injury checklist, I find these illustrations represent my persistent intellectual impairments with attention, making decisions, concentration, solving problems, understanding spoken and written instructions, doing simple math, starting or initiating, executing tasks, learning new things and tracking, hence misplacing things. I am also now very literal. Learning and naming my annoying difficulties is helping me to understand and maybe have more patience with myself when I am reminded, as I cannot retain all of this information.

Through a depression journal with my therapist and self-observations, I find I have mood swings from depression to anger to despair in this time frame. Persistent mood disorders and persistent physiological impairments abound. Very uncharacteristically, anger sometimes now results in temper outbursts that I cannot control via shouting or throwing rubber balls against the wall (encouraged by my rehabilitation team). During an angry outburst and at other times, I find I have persistent physiological indicators. In a flashback, my heart is pounding, my thoughts are racing, my pulse is rapid and my head pains intensely. Tense feelings give way to restlessness, for which I pace back and forth in my power wheelchair, up and down, up and down the hall fast, trying to get rid of some of the energy. The flashbacks invade my sleep as nightmares. Owing to these nightmares and TBI symptomatology, I have disturbed sleep. I awaken frequently during the night. It is difficult for me to fall asleep and stay asleep. Sleep is aggravated additionally by sleep apnea, causally related to the TBI. The difference between others' nightmares and mine is that when others wake up, their nightmare ends. I am still living mine. I am easily fatigued and have a considerable loss of physical strength compared to pre-TBI.

Exceptionally uncharacteristic of my determinedly independent self, at this time, I have passivity. It is deemed a persistent personality alteration. I do not speak up. I am very unaware of myself and my surroundings and have significant communication difficulties. Other alterations reveal I am also emotionally numb. Impulsiveness, which was not a part of my repertoire, causes reasons for concern and some humorous-after-the-fact purchasing incidents. Indiscreet comments are coming out as never before. I am struggling to learn to monitor them. I also persist with chronic frustration in my day-to-day struggle to get back to me.

Persistent psychological consequences of TBI are also universal with PTSD. To truly be transparent about the consequences of TBI, I am baring my soul here. In this time frame, I have developed an impaired and very negative sense of myself to the point of suicidal ideation. I have feelings of worthlessness. Feelings of depression, as well as fear and dread, alternate inside me. Everything feels like an effort. I have to make an effort just to make an effort. Discouragement abounds. I am now easily agitated and irritated. Crying keeps happening easily without an apparent cause, emotionality I did not have pre-TBI. This is leading to more feelings of discouragement, which is causing me to withdraw more into social isolation. Hypervigilance of my environment is heightened severely. Noises rattle me so that I almost fall out of my wheelchair. My startle response is extreme. I cannot form the words to express these feelings to my loved ones.

I zone out or sometimes go into my fog, a state of nothingness. I am in an altered state of consciousness. I am learning from the checklist that this is a persistent neurological problem from TBI. It is also a PTSD symptom. I have a slowed reaction time. Neurologically, I attain blurred vision and sometimes double vision, especially when I am fatigued. Sensitivities to sound and noise, in addition to light, continue. These neurological effects hinder me socially and also contribute to my further withdrawal. I find it problematic to relax.

These many impairments are magnanimous. My articulate, intellectual, adventurous, humorous persona – my old self – is gone. Who am I as a human being? It is disheartening and confusing to be unable to wrap up the functional brain impairments in a neat container and say this is what is me, what is left of me and this is where I am headed. I am spilling out and washing away without full awareness. On 4–16–10 from Rick's progress summary reports, I wrote: *I don't know what was worse – not knowing what I didn't know, or knowing that I didn't know and trying to find a way back to knowing. Or when I did not know what I did not know, or in my further awakening when I became aware that there was a great deal I no longer knew.* I was unsure and confused, a frequent happenstance.

Stages of Grief

In this third and fourth year, I find myself in Kubler-Ross's grief stages of anger and depression. In the second stage of anger, though these stages are not linear, I now become aware that my denial cannot continue. The first point of enlightenment is to know your limitations. As I reflect on these years, I recognize that I had misplaced feelings of rage. I seemed to be angry with myself, others, and God. I wondered, "How can this happen to me?" "It's not fair." "Why would God let this happen to me?" This will be fleshed out further on.

The fourth stage of Kubler-Ross's grief is depression, which I am going through during this timeframe. I am beginning to understand the certainty of death. The idea of living has no point. Things are beginning to lose meaning. I am becoming even more silent, am very sullen and do not want to be accompanied. In self-reflection and through my process journal cryptic notes, I find that I am disconnecting from things of love and affection. This action is seen as trying to avoid further trauma. It is viewed as a rehearsal for the aftermath, a kind of acceptance with emotional attachment. As indicated, it is natural to feel uncertainty, sadness, fear and regret while moving through this stage. Supposedly, showing the beginning of acceptance of the situation results from feeling these emotions, which ideally would bring the individual to the fifth stage of acceptance. This is not happening for me. My depression thickens, by which I really mean deepens. I am on a rocky road and still have not found a throughway.

7 Lost Trailways
Relationships and Loss of Identity

Post-TBI, I have lost my identity, community, stability and coherence. I am lost as a mom, sister, daughter, cousin, aunt, friend, chairwoman, committee member, therapist, speaker, civil rights advocate, poet, colleague and student. Nowhere to be found are my mind, intelligence, ease and ability to articulate, independence, capability, ground and barrier-breaking competencies, my organization and leadership proficiency and a host of other discriminating attributes.

In my stricken state, I am reminded of several poems I wrote several years after becoming disabled by paraplegia. These poems culminated into a book of poetry, *They Forgot I Had Feelings Though I Could Not Feel* (Genetti, 1992), depicting my feelings and reactions when I first became disabled, which caused a critical loss of identity. The first haiku is:

A fragile rosebud
Struggling to burst outward
In all its glory.

I am having a very difficult time relating to others. I feel very detached from people. Communicating is still markedly poor. My concept of self is diminishing, falling to pieces, completely depleting during my third year as a TBI survivor. From my journal:

I feel so removed and lonely. I have lost 'me' and I want ME back.

I found that social isolation is a broad area, which includes marginalization in multiple communities, difficulties in interpersonal relationships, difficulty in employment and the invisibility of cognitive disabilities.

DOI: 10.4324/9781003428510-11

Changes in Interpersonal Relationships

Through my research, I find that one of the domains of the post-traumatic growth concept is a change in interpersonal relationships. Some individuals improve relationships over time by having an increased compassion for others, an increased feeling of significance for family and friends, and an aspiration for more closeness in relationships. However, in the aftermath of TBI, many survivors and family members express drastic changes in their relationships with a negative impact. I am no exception. Grand challenges ensue related to a TBI survivor's social network, which include: social interaction with relatives, friends, co-workers and professional care providers. All of my trailways to social connections seem lost.

I am not alone in this predicament. I am finding that developing and maintaining meaningful relationships, family life, work and other activities of daily living are obstructed by both the cognitive and physical sequelae of TBI. Additionally, the emotional, psychological and behavioral sequelae of TBI contribute considerably more negative impact on relationships, and to further disability. I found numerous adverse coping effects with negatively associated factors of both PTG and TBI. They consist of: behavioral problems, social exclusion and isolation, burden to the family, above-average marital breakdown, poor return to work and negative appreciation of life. These add to the emotional functioning that are the new realities of adjusting to TBI.

Closest Relationships

I have a close relationship with Jay. He and I have been lifelong friends since 12 years of age. Jay is also my driver and has now taken over working as my personal assistant (PA), which he did as a backup pre-car crash. My PA had to leave soon after my accident, which complicates my situation even more. I am not capable of hiring and training someone new at this point. Jay and I look after each other even though we live independently in our own homes, Jay in New Hampshire and me here in Massachusetts. Jay lives the life of a bachelor, carefree and not on anyone's schedule. He has never married or had children. We have an awesome relationship, and although we are not significant others, we consider each other like family.

I seem to have held the more responsible role between us, using my motherly wiles. Suddenly, due to the car crash, we are thrown into a role reversal where Jay is thrust into caretaker. He physically is my closest to next of kin to jump in and help me. My Dad is also coming from New Jersey to stay for about four weeks at a time periodically, especially after my surgeries when he stays for a longer duration. Jay and I have crash-landed into a road that turns rocky as neither of us is prepared for me to be dependent on him. Our friendship endures after almost crumpling during this timeframe.

Many parts of our lives are changing. There seems to be no time for friendship, fun or leisure. I am no longer his intelligent and fun-loving companion who can handle multiple tasks times two without breaking a sweat, or an empathic listener and problem-solver. Now, here I sit with little physical mobility, and I forget what Jay just asked or told me three minutes ago. All our time is spent on my recovery and the basics of daily living, which is chaotic and frenzied. Jay has been amazing in what he is taking on. I cannot even make a decision, for instance, what I want to eat, nor even choose between two selections. Jay just makes these kinds of decisions for me now and provides me with what he thinks I need. There is no time for things I might like. There is no time to wait to see if I have a thought of what I'd like.

Complicating issues is that Jay is not a planner or caretaker, and I am not a *caretakee*. Our communication is becoming difficult. We misunderstand what each other is thinking, often causing feelings of aloneness, isolation and being overwhelmed. Frustration and stress keep appearing. We are both getting lost in this reverse relationship. We're detaching emotionally, and it is difficult to realize and adjust together. We have no time to stop and evaluate what is happening to us. We have the stress and anxiety of not knowing how long this situation is going to go on, how much better I can be and if so, when? We both need emotional support in new ways and are unavailable to each other. We both miss the me who would know what to do.

I feel my physical limitations and my needs are a heavy burden for Jay and for my father. There is a burden for caretakers. I feel like they are frustrated and mad at me often. There is also a burden for survivors to try to accept becoming "the dependent." I fight to assist while forgetting, remembering and struggling to be independent. It is difficult to know that I cannot do things by myself, and I do not want to ask for help. My physical reality is that I am still recovering from rotator cuff surgery with my right arm in a sling, and both legs are paralyzed. I have the use of only one limb, my left arm. I am finding great hardship. I have tremendous difficulty transferring my body from my wheelchair to bed or to an easy chair in the living room. I am still using a power wheelchair, which I have not perfected the art of, especially due to my eyesight, as I cannot physically wheel my manual wheelchair anymore. I bump into and mar many walls, especially going around corners, which irritates everyone. I have the most severe headaches that have not let up. The lights are too bright, yet hardly any are on. The slightest pin drop sounds like a big chunk of metal hitting the floor. It feels like my head will split open or explode.

I need assistance, support and care just to get through the day. This is very difficult for me to admit and accept. I am ambivalent, but I am very dependent after my brain injury. I move about, but everything is difficult. I need someone to help me acquire meals, to drive and accompany me to appointments, to clean and to stimulate me if around when I roll into my deep fogginess. I need someone to help resolve problems, to make decisions, read something and interpret the meaning for me and to take care of personal business. In order to live my life, I have so much dependency on a few others than at any other time in my life. I have always been self-reliant and, yes, staunchly independent since my very early teens. I have always trusted that I can take care of any of my needs on my own, and I want to.

Out of frustration, Jay has made a list of his own things I can no longer do or need help with daily:

> *the most fundamental basics of daily living, fill the dog food bins as Dee forgets, call in refills and set up her prescriptions, push her manual wheelchair for all functions outside the house. She can only do one thing at a time – one-step direction that is very limiting; can't go grocery shopping even with someone because it is overstimulating; she was a planner by nature but has great difficulty trying to plan anything including daily structure; she could advocate for anyone but now can't even for herself; time goes by and she doesn't know where it went, she never used to waste a minute; wheelchair transfer assistance; can't groom her dogs as she used to; sort or respond to mail; trouble thinking by herself – she needs someone to bounce things off of or tends to zone out; can't make her own appointments or a simple phone call; decide what to eat or when; select clothes and assist dressing; can't read the daily newspaper or keep up with current events; without appointments in her day she draws a blank for what to do so does nothing, zones out; has low stamina, low energy and attention. She has lost her creativity, sense of humor, ability to take care of her many plants, have a conversation, and basically whole future.*

Confirmation of Relationship Changes

In hindsight, through my research, I am again finding I am not alone in this struggle. Autonomy changes for many individuals with TBI in everyday life. Many survivors experience a dependence on others (e.g., next of kin) that occurs immediately after or in a short period post-injury. They also need assistance in domains including housekeeping, personal care and cognition, no matter how independent they were pre-injury. As a result, friends and families have a heavy burden placed on them, and many demonstrate an inability to cope with the TBI survivor's changes. Friends and family members detach socially and emotionally, escalating the TBI survivor's sense of alienation, which I am experiencing firsthand. Survivors are surprised by these changes and how they make them feel and behave differently in their relationships. There is a negative impact on relationships with role changes.

Spouses or partners, specifically, must often change many parts of their lives: changes in relationship roles, changes in responsibilities and challenges and changes in communication, which occur instantly and with no preparation as a result of TBI. Survivors frequently have new challenges, fears, personality traits and limitations. Significant role changes following the brain injury may characterize quite a challenge for both partners and may result in both partners feeling alone and isolated. This causes them to pull apart from their relationship. Noted is that caregiving spouses lose their major source of emotional support and companionship and other significant role changes. Decreased social opportunities and financial strains are commonly observed as well. Between 23–73% of caregivers show evidence of psychological distress. Establishing a positive environment and looking for progress in recovery, rather than how the relationship is not succeeding, is one way to improve how people feel about each other now. Jay and I ultimately are able to do that, creating an even stronger friendship than pre-TBI.

An example of a burden on relationships is a mom who reveals what it feels like to be in her caretaker parental relationship with her adult son, who sustained a TBI. In a personal story about the real truth about brain injuries, she divulges she is a writer of articles, speeches, books and presentations, and as such, has tried to bring awareness to the devastating injury of TBI. She has tried to put an optimistic twist to every piece. She writes, though, that she has stifled her real thoughts and emotions and kept her secrets hidden. She reveals that most people try to place a positive twist on its horrors. She states in reality, however, there is no silver lining.

Family

My familial relationships are strained on one side of the family and have been for many years. I do not have support or assistance from most. I was not accepted after becoming disabled, as depicted in the following poem about my family (Genetti, 1992):

They Forgot I Had Feelings

Though

I Could not Feel

They forgot I had feelings
    though I could not feel;
they wouldn't talk to me
    until I would heal.

My physical condition
    an obvious plight,
with little mobility
    turns people to fright.

They forgot I had feelings;
    they tried not to know
the stirrings inside me
    that might scare them so.

But these feelings yet unspoken
    just fester inside;
people fear they'll be broken
    if I utter one sigh.

Emotional feelings are
    held deep in my heart
but to not burden others
    I'm tearing apart.

The awful dreaded silence
    it's worse than disease;
this deadly dreaded silence
    I cannot appease.

This dreadful silence started;
it hit hard and fast
'cause people don't know how to
    let go of the past.

Some body parts feel nothing
    yet some do remain
filled with longing and yearning
    to be heard again.

When my body is enabled
    they will again speak
but there's one thing forgotten –
    will I reach that peak?

These people pretend as they
    go on day to day,
if and when my body feels
    they'll have something to say.

They're awaiting the day this
    will simply disappear
or at least until the day
    I am out of the wheelchair.

If not, I'm confined with this
    dreaded, angry fear
of speaking to people who
    just don't care to hear.

Family

    I went to a family barbecue
Ten minutes I was to stay,
    My siblings and step-siblings
All there on the same day.

    There are twelve siblings in all,
Most with children and spouses,
    Not often do I see them –
They don't visit all of our houses.

Certain houses the siblings visit
To gossip and cause pain
To the people not there –
They are selfish, hurtful and vein.

Social discrimination
Is so hard to face –
But when it's your own family
It's impossible to erase.

Going on for six years,
My siblings showing utterly no care,
They also never helped us
Due only to fear of my chair?

No more family barbecues
I was slighted most of the time,
But when they spoke, I was called "it"
Propelled aside, and treated like slime.

From the family I've been dropped
After they stabbed me in the heart,
Looking right into my face
As they shattered me apart.

(Genetti, 1992)

I also penned a wish for those family members in the following poem, but it fell on deaf ears.

A Ray of Hope

I wish for you, each member of my family,
a wish I feel a need to share.
My wish is for a ray of hope, to guide each of us
toward peace . . . understanding . . . and tranquility.

It's not something we can purchase and deliver,
or even force upon one another to accept.
If it's not something we can have at all times, hopefully
we'll be able to summon in times of desperate need.

It's knowing that somehow, we will make things better.
And it's a warm inner feeling of knowing

we've done our best, tried our hardest –
   had the strength to face the inevitable changes called "life."

And remember, life and change are in constant
   motion, happening all around
to each of us, at the same time.
   Some changes very pleasant, others very difficult.

I wish us the wisdom to understand each other
   and to accept life's incessant changes.
And the courage to be there for each other,
   to offer tender-hearted support.

I wish for us to understand each other's pain,
   to bask in each other's joys,
to be able to reach out and share the rolling waves
   in each other's lives.

I wish for us a gentle ray of hope – hugging us
   to nudge the senses into tranquil ponderance,
and to beckon appreciation and love
   for the tiny gifts bestowed in life.

(Genetti, 1992)

I am especially close with my Dad, who resides in New Jersey, and my Aunt Pat, who is also my Godmother, in Kentucky, with whom I speak daily. She shares her wisdom, listens and is inspirational in every conversation. She truly gets the old me and the new me. I have a close relationship with one sister who has acute medical issues and cousins who all live out of state. I talk with my Dad every day on the phone and he has been coming up to help, staying for four to six weeks at a time and longer during my shoulder surgeries and recovery. My Dad and I are very close. He was shocked at the drastic changes in my mind and abilities, especially my stuttering, inability to remember, and cognitive changes. He is a great help with the physical care of me, my dogs and my household, especially making home-cooked meals. I did home-cooking every day previously and find little interest in processed food, which has been a necessity. He, too, is helping with my transfers from hospital bed to wheelchair, setting up medications, washing my hair, feeding my dogs and letting them out, playing with them, doing laundry and helping me pick out clothes.

By this third year, my Dad vacillates between being sympathetic and empathetic to trying to get me to "snap out of it" and get on with my usual life. He goes from acknowledging symptoms to then trying to normalize them as many others do. For instance, Dad says, "We all have memory problems and word-finding problems, and it is due to age or tiredness," and other excuses. The problem for me is that I have all of these symptoms all of the time, day after day after day, which is exhausting and exasperating. They seem to be a package deal. It is difficult to realize this is still going on three years later. It is even more difficult to accept that it is most likely permanent, even though I continue rehab. Dad misses our philosophical, spiritual and political discussions and talks about my counseling and research work, which are so far beyond my current capacity. My literalness and lack of humor, Dad thought, would be over by now. He absolutely thought I would fully recover due to my history of sheer strength and resilience to overcome. Sometimes, he thinks I do not try hard enough. At times, Dad demands in a booming voice that I "snap out of it!" I don't remember how it happened, but I did finally come to blows with all my closest relationships. As we went through the struggles, we seemed to emerge as butterflies from their cocoons. With us were new outlooks, stronger bonds and a lightness and beauty, reminding me of the proverb, "Just when the caterpillar thought the world was over, it became a butterfly."

Friends

Initially, I had friends and just a few family members helping me out. A website is designed for all to sign up to visit me, bring meals, go to the pharmacy and other socializing or handiness with my needs. It needs organization, which is not happening at this time. Jay cannot take the lead. There is no one at the helm. I am very unaware at this time. All my thoughts and visions are but a blur. I do not want to burden others. I cannot explain myself or express what I want or need. I am disorganized in my head. I operate in extreme slow motion, with every muscle in my body aching. I do not want my community to see me in such a way. I remain silent about my plight from those wanting to help. I find it difficult to interact with people. Eventually, a few friends set up their own system of batch cooking or bringing large take-out orders for me. They separate them into three to four meals in microwaveable packages and put them into my freezer. I can then just heat the dinners in the microwave, which is immensely helpful. After a certain time, this system dwindles, though, as I am not good company for anyone.

Loneliness is very difficult to articulate. So, too, is the social desolation I have created. I found this is not uncommon, especially in women survivors of TBI. Coming much easier than conversation is small talk. I can chit-chat and fool others briefly into not knowing I have a brain injury. But as soon as I am asked a question whereupon I have to think of an answer, my plight is revealed. My brain is scrambled, and upon demand, I do not do well conversing. I stumble over words and nonsense comes out. Very slow and labored speech and thoughts not coming together quickly continue in these next third and fourth years.

In other relationships, I am trying to communicate with two of my scholarly cohorts, but I cannot keep up with the fast-paced, exciting discussions. They are speaking of pilot studies, my pilot study and books and journals we have mutually read, which I do not remember. They are trying to be supportive. My conversation timeline is stretched to about five minutes now of chit-chat before I forget. It is complicating for others. One friend is telling me she cannot bear to see me like this without my robust updates on my doctoral work. She is revealing that she does not know how to talk to me. I have never been at a loss for words on my own subject pre-brain injury. My other friend is trying to converse about Foucault, Cézanne, Freire and other authors in whose works we are both very interested. She keeps prodding me to remember. She cannot believe what I cannot remember. "Oh, sure you do," she implores. She is stunned that I cannot add to this conversation. She is clearly frustrated and looks fearful. When I speak, I still have the halt to my voice and forget my words. I forget my work that I have always been passionate about. This aches in my heart. I know it is something near and dear to me, but I cannot remember it. It is confusing trying to talk about any of this. I cannot keep up with the flow or continuity. Although I know they love me, my lack of ability to communicate scares them away.

Impact of relationships

This is my whiny moment. Without even knowing, friends and family minimize my small successes and discount my great effort to compensate for my losses each day. They claim to know what my brain injury is like. They say they have the same symptoms – forgetfulness, word-finding, inability to express themselves, even my fatigue and then reply that it happens with age or other reasons to excuse my symptoms away. They react with baffledness to my excitement over seemingly small and, to them, trivial, independent successes. I do not know how to make new, equal relationships, as I realize the person my friends are looking for does not live here anymore. I am no longer the same outgoing, funny or witty person they once knew. Could anyone love and accept the new me "as is?"

The number of lost friends, days lost to exhaustion, events missed out on, conversations avoided are but a few examples of my lost trailways leading to isolation. I leave the TV and stereo off as I need quiet – no noise or stimulation. I am dropping out or being dropped off of most of my community service committees and commissions. I am very alone. I realize reflectively that I also encourage it. This is remarkably against my character. I am shutting people out. I do not want to speak with anyone on the phone, or have visitors, or go out. With my halted stutter, slow rate of speech, and truncated thoughts, my small circle of family and friends are missing and misinterpreting the meaning of what I am trying to say. It takes so much energy to speak, and I cannot increase my low volume to interrupt and explain my point. When I do try to speak up, I have a tendency to spit out any words that will come, many of which are inadequate to make sense. Or I talk all around the subject without the capability of getting to the point – verbose, and by the end, I forget what I am saying. People keep getting frustrated with me. Conversation is futile. It hurts deeply and creates frustration in me, too, which hampers connections. Having to exert extreme energy output, my chest sinks in and my shoulders roll forward in a slump, my head feels so heavy and my mind and body crave sleep. I feel spent/used up just from the thought of talking on the phone. I have depression, more isolation and dire loneliness. I feel I am seen as wholly incompetent.

FYI

By looking through a wider lens in my research, I find that not hearing from friends, co-workers and extended family members are frequent complaints of TBI survivors. They become aware that their phone calls, e-mails and other forms of communication are left unanswered. In my case, I am not even responding to or reaching out to others. A great number of survivors, even when spending much time with family members or friends, find themselves feeling alone.

I find that in their personage before the TBI, the survivor may have felt pride. But they may now feel sad and frustrated when asked to step aside, which is exactly what I am experiencing. Uncertainty and frustration take place during the adjustment phase, which may cause criticism between family members. People close to the survivor may not understand the need for all the changes. I find friends and family members may need to be educated about brain injury and the changes that occur. I am learning about these changes in therapy with Rick, especially through reading the book *Over My Head* (Osborn, 1998), a doctor's experience of TBI and recovery that is articulate and easy to read (for others). I am unable to describe/ define traumatic brain injury, so I refer my closest family members and friends to the book. What an amazing relief as each reads the book. It eases their frustrations with me. They get to see the whole picture and how these many, many symptoms affect daily life holistically. It is still, however, hard to accept for all of us. I am writing this book to articulate to survivors, family members, caretakers and friends the many symptoms of TBI and demonstrate how they are exhibited and expressed through multiple relationships. Hopefully, it will bring a sigh of relief by understanding the underlying dynamics. It is much easier to deal with problems and behaviors once we understand them.

Stigma

When I become able to reflect a bit, more than three years post-trauma, I become very aware of the oppression and stigma out in the community. As I spread my wings more fully, I find that oppression spreads almost universally. People look down on me. I know I have limitations of functioning and that I do not shine as brightly as I did. But – I am still higher functioning than many with TBI, as I am told. I am treated as if I have no authority and no understanding. People question my ability to live independently, as I have been living since my children have grown. I am reminded of the poem I wrote in the late 1980s called *The Sub-Humans*. It was written when I, and a few people who looked like me, first ventured out into the community in our wheelchairs. It was not a typical sight to see, especially since most community spaces were not wheelchair accessible. People gasped, pulled their children away and crossed to the other walkway to avoid us.

With my slowed speech, sometimes totally blank for a minute or two, or saying something off-topic, people look at me as though I have either two heads or just one half of one. Some people quickly step back from me, while others lean down and talk loudly and more slowly into my face, enunciating every word. This attacks my auditory system and still does not produce the right response. My speech freezes or stutters. A majority of people, however, ignore me. They look above my head to finish their talk with whoever is with me. It is as though I am not even here. This also happens with family members. No one seems to be patient enough or willing to wait to understand what I am trying to say.

Increased Awareness

I start to realize, on some level, there are a lot of things I will never be able to do on my own anymore. I am realizing I need people's help – in fact, I am realizing I am dependent on help. I am my own worst enemy. I am trying desperately to be independent while not being able to remember what it is I am trying to do, unsuccessfully. And that I am not physically capable nor cognitively able to do. This is making relationships more difficult. For the ones I need to depend mostly on, it is crushing me. I am feeling a multitude of frustration thrown at me constantly. I am experiencing the tiredness of others as resentment towards me. There *are* people who want to help me. But, it has been feeling to me like they are taking away/yanking away the last bit of control I have left. It is hard to reconcile all my losses. When I finally do let go of enough control, it is a relief to realize I do have the relationships and assistance.

I found that over time, as the survivor recovers, this dependence can decrease and the experience of independence can increase. Further, the feeling of independence is vitally important for the process of recovery after TBI. For the survivor, it influences the experience of self-confidence and self-esteem. Common areas of social functioning difficulty for persons with brain injuries include a lack of social support, lack of access to services (specifically public transportation for me as I cannot follow directions independently), loss of power and control and social devaluation.

Some of my thoughts pulled from my journal during these times represent my awareness of relationships:

> *"Everyone trying to finish sentence – cut me off – no patience to hear – have no particular day-end value. My isolation;" "people treat as I mentally impaired;" "I only feel confliction with no clarity – relationships dwindle rapidly;" "feel can't count on anyone – these devastating times – so alone, unaccompanied, isolated – I detaching to others seem vacant – I want people hear me – to get me – feel my horror – know what going inside head – bad thoughts;" "have a struggle to get old self out – in few minutes*

forget what trying;" "can represent fraction of who I was/am – still not sure if I say who I was or who I am;" "am a void with nothing to give back – I didn't know."

In spite of my coming to the realization of how much I have lost, I continue my work with Rick. I am developing a strong bond, striving gruelingly to write and to get back to my dissertation. I have my amazing doctoral committee members cheering me on for continued and fullest recovery. They continue to support my struggle and show their faith in me, which motivates me. I have strong relationships and significant support from my professional team, who have brought me through the first two years and are carrying me through this third and most difficult year, especially my therapist. I also have my pastoral minister, who has been coming here every Sunday for many years. He plays a key role in my recovery spiritually, especially when I lose faith. I am missing many relationships, but I have a small support system of people who matter. Maybe the end of this trailway will not be lost but will connect me to a new path.

8 Finding a Footpath
Rehabilitation and My Life Coach

My weekly routine revolves around my rehabilitation treatment. Having the stamina to carry out only one appointment in a day, I often have two events scheduled. I am so fatigued. I am trying to find places to sleep for a few minutes in between appointments in order to cognitively be present. Speech-language-cognitive therapy (ST) is happening with Rick two days a week. I am attending physical therapy (PT) with Kate two days a week for my rotator cuff, head and neck injuries, which are still significant. Since having the shoulder surgery twice now, I can still use my arm just minimally. I am coping with much pain. I need assistance with my painful at-home exercises and the complicated shoulder apparatus that positions and stretches my shoulder in various positions. My physical condition is continuing to take more power and independence away from me.

One day a week, I am attending occupational therapy (OT) with Susan. Our focus is on compensatory strategies for shoulder and arm alternative ways of performing activities of daily living. Such activities, for example, include showering and dressing. We are investigating cognitive skills to improve activities, such as cooking. I persistently fail with these skills. I do not have the attention and wherewithal to boil an egg and remove it safely from the pan and stove. For some reason, I continue to check the temperature by sticking my fingers into the water so quickly that I don't have time to think about it. It burns. And I forget to check on what is currently cooking after two minutes.

I am attending assistive technology therapy (AT) with Rachael one day a week for durations with breaks in between. I am learning and relearning compensatory strategies. It is not going very well. I repeatedly forget several months after I relearn. Sometimes, I feel like I am banging my head against the wall, but I desperately want to improve, so I persist. Assistive tools I am trying to employ include: my tape recorder, environmental controls, my speech recognition

DOI: 10.4324/9781003428510-12

program on my computer, my dictation program "Dragon Naturally Speaking" and several other high and low technology supports. I can only work with one device at a time.

I am seeing Ellie in psychotherapy one day a week. Flashbacks continue to be a major intrusion and other symptoms of PTSD, depression and, further on, anger. Appointments with Dr. Bob, my PCP, continue every three weeks. He is my overall medical coordinator, who follows and directs my care. Dr. C is my physiatrist-rehabilitation doctor at the Spaulding Rehabilitation Hospital TBI clinic. I receive trigger point injections and acupuncture in my head, neck and shoulder every three weeks, and he follows up on my TBI progress. Most of my therapies take place at Spaulding Rehabilitation Hospital. I have gone from seeing clients/patients daily to being a client/patient daily.

In this timeframe, I am rendering progress! I will advance to 30 minutes of uninterrupted work, attempting to focus, concentrate and catch myself if I wander. I am discovering strategies to pull myself back into awareness if I can capture that I am off somewhere in my fog. This strategy is a leading goal for my self-awareness. My days blend into the weekend. Although, on Sunday mornings, I have a weekly visit with Robert, my Eucharistic Minister and spiritual advisor, for about two hours. We partake in the recitation of a prayerful mass and communion. We engage in a spiritual conversation in conjunction with the day's gospel. We then follow up with a catch-up conversation on each other's lives. I have known Robert for well over ten years, as he also taught Catechism lessons to my sons. In the latter part of this third-year post-injury, Robert has penned his opinion on how I am doing in my recovery. Trying to be very gentle, knowing that I will be reading this, he writes:

> *Dee has lack of concentration in verbal conversation. She has hesitation in verbal responses, pausing between words. Enunciation of words are somewhat slurred on occasion. She occasionally has a loss of focus. Dee is not always alert or as quick with response. She shows visible expressions and signs of depression and fatigue. She has obvious organizational deficiency, and forgetfulness.*
>
> *Dee is not the same vibrant, enthusiastic, upbeat person she was before her latest auto accident. Her functional abilities are <u>certainly not</u> what they used to be. Her direction in her life has been substantially altered if not ended. Her whole life was devoted to continuing education to help others but has hit a wall which is causing her depression and negative moods.*

Robert still encourages me weekly, helping to lift and enlighten my spirit.

Discovering My Life Coach: MY Mentor

I want to introduce you in more depth to R. Richard Sanders, M.S, CCC-SLP, my senior Speech Language Pathology Advanced Clinical Specialist at Spaulding Rehabilitation Hospital. Rick influences my life in noteworthy ways and has come to be my awesome mentor. A number of TBI survivors have a need for betterment and a more satisfying life from the emotional pain and upheaval they now endure. Maybe all TBI survivors do, but not all are able. With Rick, I am able to do something about my status post-injury. According to the Brain Injury Association of Massachusetts (BIA-MA), affected individuals with TBI may, with a redefinition of realistic goals, be able to learn compensatory skills that can enable them to return to a productive life. Productive life, however, is undefined. This is big news since many professionals are of the opinion that it is not fixable. Rick works primarily with people with acquired brain injuries, with those who are considered high functioning. This is the category I fall under. With Rick, I am finding a footpath after the lost trailways and dead ends on my rocky road.

Rick is situated as a specialist in cognition. A measure of his patients are post-graduates, with at least one being a published author. Our goal is to improve my speech, language and cognitive deficits. In particular, we will concentrate on those that affect my reading and writing, which touch every aspect of my life. I enter Spaulding Rehabilitation Hospital at a very basic level, not remembering enough information to write in a full sentence.

Rick stands very tall. He is a lean, distinguished-looking gentleman with a soft, even-toned voice and a calming demeanor. He projects warmth and friendliness while maintaining professionalism. As my mentor, Rick imparts his skills, principles, wisdom and perspectives that are making an impact on my life in this cultural group of TBI, PTSD and cognitive disabilities. Rick illuminates my path of uncertainty. His mentoring shapes and socializes the ability in disability of brain injury culture for me. As a mentee, Rick shares knowledge of my new cultural group, slowly. He keeps me focused on my overall goal to achieve scholarly writing and to return to my doctoral program. This, to me, means to write my dissertation. I lost my greatest abilities. They were my outstanding memory, exceptional writing ability and public speaking. I had a photographic memory, for which I retained material without exertion. I automatically memorized: numbers, especially phone numbers, names and addresses, books and reading materials and items that I wrote down. I could also remember things auditorily. I could remember verbatim after hearing lectures, interviews and many times by listening in general. This gift has been essential after my eyesight dropped to legal blindness.

Let me bring you into my first meeting with Rick. Jay has driven my then Service Dog, Othello, and me to Spaulding Rehabilitation Hospital in Boston. I still have my halting, stuttering, very slow, low-volume voice as I struggle to tell Rick my needs. I am pulling out half-thoughts and fragments from the whirlpool of images and ideas that have begun racing and swirling in my brain. The articulate me inside is SCREAMING to be let out, but I do not know how to reach her. I have come armed with support material. I am flailingly trying to inform Rick that I am an intelligent person inside, ready and willing to do the work. Only a garbled salad of words splutters out. I am not accepting my fate as Kathy advised. I sit here before Rick in my wheelchair, my right arm painfully dangling from the shoulder surgery. I draw out my professional resume along with my five-page community service resume of over 20 years. I have resorted to carrying these papers around with me. In case that would not be enough, I also produce my stellar and professional references, including those for entrance into my MA and PhD degree programs. AND I bring my 32-page "Biological Bases of Behavior" research paper I wrote on the neurobiological distinction between PTSD and Major Depressive Disorder (MDD). I am waving these papers in the air and stammering, "This is me, the real me – not this me [I point to myself]. I want to get back to her."

I feel extremely strongly that I need Rick's help and that it is essential for him to know who I really am in order to get me back to me. Few people "get" that I was/am an intelligent being desperately trying to be so again. I do carry my resumes and references to demonstrate to people, mainly medical professionals, who I am and where I expect to be. Professionals are usually quite astonished if they take a look. They respond to me in a more positive way, which is stigmatizing to the majority in this culture. It is my desperate way to appeal for higher aspirations. Everyone *should be* seen for their highest potential. I see this issue as a part of my future course of advocacy for TBI survivors. Rick's written goal for me is to relearn writing with the following objectives:

> *to be able to write in full thoughts and sentences, stay focused on the paragraph and be able to decipher the main and supporting sentences, both in writing and in reading comprehension.*

I am very disorganized in my head, in all my surroundings and with the notes I am trying to keep for therapy sessions. My house now looks like my brain feels – scrambled. In Rick's mentorship, he is helping to organize me and my daily living predicaments twice each week. My life schedule revolves around my medical appointments and therapies, daily homework for speech-language-cognitive therapy, 20–30 minutes at a time, and physical therapy exercises. Rick is an inspiration and my window to the outside world. We are developing a relationship built on trust and mutuality, which evokes positive growth in me. He is listening as I hesitate in my halted and slowed speech pattern and encouraging me to continue to speak. Rick is adept at reining me in when I go out of focus and off on tangents. This, unfortunately, occurs quite frequently. Rick causes me to feel more like a peer than a brain-damaged person with nothing important to contribute to my environment. I feel hopeful. He influences me to believe in myself, even though I do not know who I am.

In this timeframe, as my mentor, Rick endows me slowly with education, particularly pertaining to traumatic brain injury. This benefits me in understanding some of my confusing and exasperating symptoms. At times, Rick supplies me with a resource or, most recently, refers me to a resource. By referring me, Rick wants me to try out my research capabilities to look it up myself. Sometimes it works; many times, it does not. I did not realize for several years how repetitive Rick is, week after week after week, teaching me the same thing over again. It is new to me each time. With Rick's patience, he does not tell me. The finding came whilst reading back in my Rick-session journal notes that I have filed in different but similar folder names. They are scattered in many places on my computer. I do not remember where I put them, and I apparently do not have just one file for each subject.

Rick is engaging me in the same capacity as a student. Believing in me, Rick is giving me no false hope as to whether I will regain the skills necessary to write my dissertation. Delivering feedback to me, Rick expresses that I am extraordinary in my diligence. Further, he replies that he is surprised by my courage and tenacity to pursue and to continue to accomplish skills in the language, cognitive and writing arenas. Coaching me on how to frame my feelings into words, Rick is also teaching me to generate an action plan, which I call a *Rick list*. I am working on and generating many Rick lists. Rick is rising to be my life coach. He is showing me how to master undertakings or at least gain new knowledge for that which no longer comes naturally. Rick is helping me to attempt to organize, one task at a time. We are developing structures and systems for dealing with time and life-solving problems.

With Rick's guidance, I am starting to perceive there is life after brain injury. He is steering me down the slippery slope, engaging with me in my quest to evolve and return to my doctoral program. Consequently, we will also work on social endeavors. Rick will introduce me to the reading of a book about a doctor with a TBI and will encourage me to reach out to her. He will recommend a support group and, further on, will invite me to speak at engagements for future language therapists who will work with survivors of acquired brain injuries.

As an advanced clinical speech therapist, Rick is providing me with skills and information, but a mentor does more – they also confer something that causes you to believe in yourself. Rick just disclosed to me that when he was a Teaching Assistant, he had a professor who believed in him. He showed a personal interest and treated Rick like a human being. Rick related that those acts have always stayed with him. That is exactly how Rick makes *me* feel! Orchestrating the way to finding myself, or the new me, Rick is instrumental in helping me develop self-worth. At the same time, he is helping me try to shed the shame and stigmatization I feel to my core. Even with an undefined identity, I have kept my strong aspiration and sense of urgency to get the intelligent me back. With the general public learning about TBI in our returning soldiers from Iraq and Afghanistan, the stigma of having a mental disorder relating TBI to mental derangement is slowly changing. Rick is influencing me to believe there is no shame or stigma in having a head injury. Rather, Rick insists, it is society that has to change their viewpoints.

After realizing I had lost my persona and coherence, I find Rick is my compass. He is directing me toward healing and resurgence. Rick is helping me on a path to finding a sense of myself and new values to at least rebuild a life that is tolerable. His hope is for me to move up on Maslow's (1954) Hierarchy of Basic Needs – again, and thrive. My physiological needs are met. I do have to go through the redevelopment of subsequent safety, then ascend to belonging, next onto self-worth and self-respect, followed by self-actualization. This will be the rebirth of who I am. I have to redevelop all of my previous well-developed stages as I seek to satisfy my need for fulfillment.

Rick is guiding me through my foggy maze, which is slow-going. He is a benevolent, consistent presence. Teaching me how to think and function with success again through cognitive and metacognitive skills training is a reconstruction that is so valuable. I do not even have the words to describe what it means to me. Rick is also very honest, which is not easy at times. It is two years that we have been working together. I need Rick to state my prognosis. My health insurance just decided I am not progressing rapidly enough, even though my measurable progress continues. They terminated my coverage. This news is almost unfathomable. I need Rick's tutelage! Rick helps me to arrange to continue to see him, though, as a private patient at Spaulding Rehabilitation Hospital. I cannot afford to pay much privately. I can barely afford the expense of meeting with Rick once every two weeks. This alters everything! I now proceed from seeing him eight times a month to seeing him two to three times a month. I am set in turmoil! I feel lost, stranded, abandoned and disordered in a substantial way again. It will take an inordinate amount of time to restructure my life again.

I met with the Massachusetts Rehabilitation Commission regarding possible assistance. They express that they will consider vocational assistance to include payment for my speech-language-cognitive treatment. The case manager informs me she just needs Rick to say that I can finish a dissertation and will be gainfully employed afterward. Rick is not going to do that. He reasons that he cannot predict where anyone can get to or what the therapy outcome will be. Therefore, I do not get the assistance. Rick, though, assures me he will continue working with me as earnestly as we have been. He states this will continue for as long as we both feel I am making progress toward my goal. Rick's positive presentation motivates me. I have a full sense that I can count on Rick, especially in times of trouble, even though this case did not go my way. He encourages me to keep on going against difficult odds. I am making the road ahead for me. Rick reiterates that he believes in me no matter where that road goes. These are feelings I can hold onto.

I tremendously value my relationship with Rick. Through him, I am developing a sense of closeness with others. It is happening first as I relate to the main character, a fellow TBI traveler, in the book we read in therapy *Over My Head* (Osborn, 1998). It again happens with more medical professionals at Spaulding Rehab that I need to rely on. Ultimately, I will meet with and relate to others with similar injuries and sequelae like mine on a speaker panel of TBI survivors. The wheels on my wheelchair seem firmly placed on this footpath.

9 Unearthing Stepping Stones
Learning to Read and Write

The basic goals for reading and writing begin with "grasping words." I am learning under Rick's auspices. I am beginning to gain a number of new strategies for my significant word retrieval troubles. For instance, when I cannot find the word that I am searching for, I move through the alphabet letter by letter. Sometimes, if I hear the first letter, I can get the word. I have brain exercise worksheets for finding a new word. The worksheets encourage the use of my brain to process information, concentrate and otherwise toggle my brain to work. An example of finding a new word is to change a letter and then turn it into a new word. For instance, I start with the word *make,* and I change it to *b*ake, *c*ake, *f*ake, *l*ake, etc. I have to select a letter and then make it a word with *ake* in alphabetical order, which is challenging for me. Another exercise for words is to construct compound words by methodically going through the alphabet by consonant letters and then adding vowels in order. The intent is to jog my mind into finding the other half of the word. Hampering this effort is that I am quite literal now, not abstract, just concrete. This causes more rigidity in thinking.

In this third- and fourth-year timeframe, I am learning how to turn words into fragments and then into sentences. I am working on thinking in complete thoughts. For an exercise, I am reading short three-sentence stories. Following, I am taking notes that I think are adequate. They keep turning out to be cryptic – in bullet points with just a few words. As it turns out, when I read them back, there are not enough words to flesh out the bullet points into a meaningful idea. It is like I scattered some stones and wheeled onto one, but it does not connect to another. There is no real path there. With Rick, I try to put the stones in a row or in a line, so I can actually wheel down the path and get somewhere. Schooling me on sentence structure, I am learning to add who did what, when, where, why or

DOI: 10.4324/9781003428510-13

in the old way we learned in English class subject-verb-object. I lose information trying to think of all of that, as I cannot hold onto every word or thought. I wonder, in a summary note to Rick from Rick's files, as I have to write important notions down (it is edited with Rick for completeness), "*Is it better to write a sentence and lose a lot of it, or better to just get thoughts down even if they are half thoughts?*" I practice doing either, and I struggle to do both.

My working memory is still greatly compromised. I can read a sentence and decode the words, but then I forget what immediately preceded it. I have a déjà vu feeling from when I was a child reading in the dark with a penlight under the sheets. I would be able to get a word before and a word that came next. That was the extent of my focus. I am increasingly able to get the sentence before and sometimes anticipate the sentence next, but anything larger is difficult.

Writing a sentence involves looking at the words I have written on my computer. Subsequently, I have to realize that I have a non-sentence and further try to expand it to render a complete sentence. When I think I've arranged it, I take a break and roll away from my computer. I wheel back with a clearer head. After reading and editing and re-reading and re-editing, checking subject-verb-object and who, what, where and when, I finally finish the sentence. My feelings are either depleted by the agony of the length of time to complete the sentence or I feel very triumphant that I am able to construct it, and sometimes I feel both. Onto sentence two – I hope. Writing one good sentence can occupy six or more broken-up hours of 15–30 minutes a session over several days. Somehow, it seems like when I can compose the perfect grammatical, full sentence, I will be cured. Of course, this constitutes no sense, but it did not seem to matter to me. This undertaking consumes a whole week, all seven days, to write a small three-sentence paragraph . . . and then I start the process over again.

A sample of sentences that includes my word-finding problems, writing the wrong word and sentence structure problems is seen clearly in my session homework pages for Rick. These sentences were already proofread by me without my seeing a problem:

> *It does not later; Write incomplete thoughts and then I will sink and complete thoughts; When reading stop when fe summary; I could totally relate to, struggling with the same times of problems – primary goal get been to doctoring work; Write and the formal for each sentence, explain my thoughts and writing whole sentence just fragments I forget what talking.*

In this timeframe, I am using more words to flesh out a sentence, but they are not always decipherable. I have to use my strategies to check for each word and each sentence grammatically – it uses extreme labor.

Learning organization of material is evident through my draft exercises. I am listening to short news stories on NPR on the web. I began with two to three-minute stories, unable to answer any questions. As I increase retention, I am expanding my memory and ability to take in new information. In this fourth year, I am reaching a step further. I am endeavoring to write briefly a synopsis of the story to practice writing after listening. This will heighten information coming in and hopefully give me the ability to write a summary. It is akin to writing a summary of a conference I would attend for my professionalism. I need to be able to take in enough information when listening to or reading new material. Then I need to process it in my head and finally put it back out on paper. It will be vital to writing my dissertation. I expand my listening capacity and ability in this timeframe from two to three minutes to 30 minutes at a sitting! What an amazing achievement by the end of the fourth year post-TBI.

Note-taking is another lesson I am learning that has its challenges. I have a thought, hold a pen, and by the time my thought goes from my brain to the end of my pen, I forget what I want to write. Rick's new strategy for me is to keep my computer on all day. Therefore, when I have a thought, I can type it instantaneously. Arthritis and injury to my right hand render that to be more difficult. The next strategy is to use Dragon Naturally Speaking, a voice recognition program for my computer. Training with and having it recognize my voice, speech patterns and vocabulary and learning the commands is exceedingly challenging. Recognition is flawed and complicated for me. I am successful one minute but unsuccessful the next. Years go by before I can use it effectively, working with Rachael in assistive technology. It does not happen in this time frame. I am conquering my stuttering, though, which is a factor for speech recognition. Another factor is my difficulty in thinking on demand, which complicates usage. And I keep forgetting the commands – frustrating!

Rick decides to refer me to assistive technology for several other reasons, as well. A great one is to relearn how to organize my computer. My *Rick files* are in many places because I keep forgetting where I put them and what I name our session notes and my homework. The many files are on my computer, in my office and maybe in my kitchen. When I go to retrieve a file, nothing sounds familiar, so I start a new one. The third reason is to refresh my memory by using my speech program, JAWS, on my computer. The program reads the screen to me as I type, word by word, line by line, or all the way through the page, to accommodate my low vision. I continually forget the keystrokes and commands to operate the program and set up a page.

A Few More Rick Strategies

Rick is teaching me step-by-step directions for many instances. While he is dictating, I am taking notes on my computer. Rick is confirming I have written enough words to make sense by surveying my screen frequently. We are formulating itinerary lists into words, especially ones slated for my medical professionals: what and how to say what I need to communicate my thoughts. I still do not transmit enough information to my doctors. I am very discouraged when I leave. No wonder I get overlooked as just another brain-damaged patient!

Part one of a new effective compensatory strategy is writing notes to myself and posting them in plain view. Then, I have to act on them!! as part two. I write in large print with a thick red Sharpie with few words so I can catch sight of them. I line them up under my Optilec, a reading machine that magnifies text up to 60%. This is actually helping with my productivity and organization! Rick is a big fan of Post-It notes and lists. I often show up missing something for each of my sessions. Rick assists me with making a list. He then firmly reminds me to post it on a cabinet near my back door. I innovatively call it my "going-out-the-door list." It does take me time, however, to actually look at it. It takes even longer to eventually ask my driver to gather the items with me (backpack, computer, power supply, tape recorder, worksheets or summaries, cell phone, sunglasses and water).

Rick and I are establishing strategies for activities of daily living (ADLs). I am trying to use a notebook appointment planner. I try a calendar on my computer, but I cannot remember the few steps to access and use it. My life is getting scheduled and listed with strategies for taking care of my home: a plan for paying bills by means of a calendar, several ways of compiling a shopping list, microwave cooking steps for heating up food and contacting Stacy at the bank to set up partial online banking. This sounds wonderfully organized! It will take several years for me to set up and re-set up and then to follow each strategy, even with the assistance of others at my home.

Two Break-through Events

In this fourth year post-TBI, I can still only hold one step in my head at a time. Multitasking has been long gone. Rick calmy and methodically helps me to follow one step and then the next without getting overwhelmed. Rick tries a strategy to relate my speech-language training to my doctoral work. We utilize a recording from one of my clinical sessions from my pilot research project. The idea is to attempt to transcribe it. As Rick is working with me, he ensures that I write enough words in a step before moving to the next, which he is dictating to me. From my session notes:

Focus on one step at a time and the steps are:

1. Find the recording file to transcribe, take a breath.
Onto step 2. Listen for two minutes all the way through for two minutes, breathe.
Next step is 3. Go back to the beginning of the two minutes.
Step 4. Listen phrase by phrase of the two minutes and speak each phrase for dictation using Dragon Dictate. Repeat until the phrase is transcribed.
Step 5. Check the Dragon text.
Step 6. Have two minutes transcribed by next week.

This task is actually a monumental event for me. I have a one-hour tape with multiple voices to convert. Rick is instilling in me a most important endeavor. It is to notice when I get overwhelmed and then stop before I glaze over. In my glazed state, my mind shuts down. I practice, but two minutes takes weeks for me to transcribe. I persevere with the transcription over the lengthy span of seven months, but not alone. I do it with assistance from Rachael in AT. By striking the keys on my computer for the commands to go back and forth from the text to the tape recording, Rachael facilitates this effort. I forget the phrase between alternating from speech (the recording which is on my computer) and the text page (on my computer) to which I am dictating. Rachael is also relaying the dictation and format commands that I just cannot retain. The words *can't* or *cannot* were never in my vocabulary pre-TBI. This is very tedious. But I did finally finish it! From my journal:

it is so tiring being me every minute of every day – would love a break for even one whole day.

And further in my journal:

> *Every day moving on way too slow and not have steady. Every day –*
> *a new day all over again, a new challenge.*

Rick stresses to me that there *is* new life after TBI. However, it is not your own or the one you lost. I lost my old life, but I am still trying to connect to it, not just replace it. I found a bit of myself! From my journal:

> *I rediscovered color – purple skirt – light aqua tee – violet blue*
> *blouse – wondered where clothes been to wear – haven't see usual*
> *color schemes – right there closet – put on today – yes – I look like me!*

10 Road to Recovery
Beginning of Self-Discovery

The road to recovery is steep, long and winding. I still bump into frequent roadblocks and get my wheels caught on stumps. At this time, I am finding my self-concept is diminishing, feeling so un-individualistic and lonely. I feel like no one understands me, or the magnitude of my losses or what I am trying to overcome and possibly to accept. In hindsight reflection, and through my research, I am finding the individual self is created through the culture, as one finds others in their place in the community. I realize there is a feeling that draws us to others at our level. When TBI survivors meet another survivor on the road, they find solace and camaraderie. This is especially true with those who are at the same functioning level of their injury impairments.

As a TBI survivor, an important part of my daily routine now centers around fatigue and rest periods. These and other new cultural behaviors and routines are not always synchronized with the rhythms of the broader society. They are patterned routines of life reflecting those from the culture in which I now participate. Through reflection and examination of records, I see how I begin to realize my new TBI culture. I am trudging down a new path in this fourth year post-TBI, and I am not sure how to navigate it. A poem I penned in the 1980s, after the spinal cord injury, comes to mind:

The Upside-Down Turtle

The upside-down turtle
his hard shell underneath
is struggling to be mobile
but can only grit his teeth.

He rocks back and forth
trying to roll from side to side

DOI: 10.4324/9781003428510-14

but he still cannot do it
and now he's losing his pride.

He needs some assistance
but no one seems to know
how to help him back to standing;
they don't help him so.

They poke him and prod him
responding with a stare
then they send him away
for another one to bear.

So, he stretches to pull forward
using all of his might;
he pushes and he pulls
every day and every night.

Alas, he starts to give up
after using all he could expend
for he forgot, you see,
that turtles just can't bend.
(Genetti, 1992)

Learning a New Lifestyle

Rick introduces me to the book *Over My Head – A Doctor's Own Story of Head Injury from the Inside Looking Out* (Osborn, 1998) by Claudia Osborn, MD. It is to be used as a tool for learning to write and for reading comprehension. The book is also my introduction to the TBI culture. I learn many months in the future from now how to make a Venn diagram to compare and contrast our lives/narratives, which is how I was able to write this self-discovery chapter.

Rick is giving me a template for taking notes while reading this narrative story. To expand my thinking and comprehension, Rick is describing a method of Predict-Read-Prove. I am to fill in the following information for each segment that I read, which begins with only two to three sentences – my working memory limit. Write the chapter title or number; the setting (where and when in just a few words); main characters involved; action or plot summary of what I just read in one to three lines; and then a one-sentence prediction or question for what might happen next. Then, I am to read the

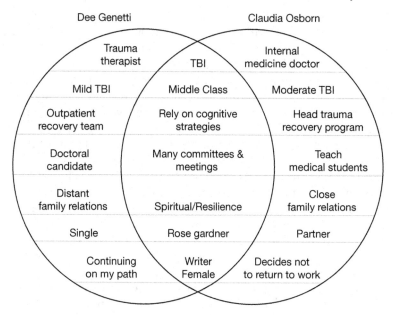

Figure 10.1 Venn Diagram

next section. Next, reread and pay attention to see if I can prove my prediction. The ability for forward-thinking to formulate a prediction or question is very challenging. Remembering enough of what I read to prove right or wrong is also a trial. I still write a few words, but not enough to construct a whole or meaningful idea. It is improving. Eventually, when I am able to read a paragraph or a whole page, Rick additionally has me write a response to either say how I feel about the content or critique Claudia. This happens much further than halfway through the book.

Contrasts and Comparisons

It is a bit disconcerting reading *Over My Head* (Osborn, 1998) here in my blue reclining chair that I transferred into from my wheelchair in my living room. Othello, my black lab service dog, is lying in a tight ball on a rug in front of the fireplace, with shiny brass doors and arms made of bricks built-in on each side, with slate slabs atop. He looks like a Currier and Ives postcard. The brass lamp with the scalloped linen shade on the Queen Anne table beside me emits a moderate amount of light, enough for me to see my computer by which to read/watch without affecting my light sensitivity. Perched on my maxi-length purple embroidered cotton skirt is a pillow that sits squarely on my lap. On top is my laptop with my speech processor. It is reading my book name and chapter title to me. A glass of water sits on the table beside a tall white vase with red roses from my rose garden. This is an example of short descriptive writing exercises that I learn to do in the future in order to prepare my mind for thinking.

As I contemplate, I am realizing I connect with Dr. Claudia Osborn through our common experience. We have very different accidents/ introductions into the TBI disability culture. Claudia is hit by a car head-on while riding her bicycle. She is knocked unconscious for an undisclosed amount of time. Claudia wakes up in the hospital emergency room and refuses to be admitted. She goes home with her significant other. The car I was in was hit by a truck, knocking me unconscious briefly. I was taken by ambulance to the hospital emergency room and, after several hours, I went home accompanied by Jay and my service dog, Othello. I plan to care for myself, as Othello and I live alone. Claudia's TBI is more severe than mine – moderate severity. Our programs for rehabilitation recovery are different but with many parallels. I realize that she is my first TBI survivor peer, high functioning like me. As well, her TBI survivor cohorts in her recovery program are TBI survivors vicariously. They are enlightening me about life with a traumatic brain injury. We all share many of the same beliefs, values, attitudes and experiences. We share an incredible bond of feeling and knowing what nobody else can who does not have a brain injury, that of knowing from the inside looking out.

It is taking me a year and a half to read this small paperback book of 232 pages. As I struggle, I then grow through each of its chapters of only about ten pages. The book begins with Claudia, who is very tired constantly and has poor memory. She is forgetting things, including what she is trying to do currently. She tries to go to work. She cannot understand the mail. She knows the words, but they do not make sense together. I am finding one of my own – Claudia, in my new sub-culture of TBI. I have an inquiry as to how Claudia will get back to practicing, and how I will – she as a teaching doctor and me as a therapist and PhD candidate – her patients and her students, my clients and my studies.

Claudia enters one of the top rehabilitation facilities for TBI, the Head Trauma Program of the Rusk Institute of Rehabilitation Medicine (HTP) in New York City. She begins an outpatient program nine months after her accident. Claudia moves to NYC from Detroit for the duration. Her sole purpose and focus, she believes, is to get better and get back to work immediately following this five month program. She is adamant, no matter what anyone says to her. In this group program of 12 students with traumatic brain injuries, each member also has a coach/mentor/guide to help them with their individual needs. They attend this program five days a week for five hours with a break for lunch. My individual rehabilitation program is also outpatient, which I begin right away. My program adds necessary individual therapy components as they become necessary. My sessions are between 45 and 60 minutes long, on different days and with breaks in between – much less intense.

We have contrasting relational support systems, which we both value tremendously. Claudia has a large support system, including familial support from her partner Marcia and her mother, who visits her periodically for long sprints of time and talks on the phone. She also has her stepfather, grandmother and other family members. Claudia has a number of friends who are a second close support system outside of this circle. Claudia lives with her partner, Marcia, and is fully independent prior to her accident. She has the support of her 11 cohorts, team coaches and head coach/mentor. Some of the advantages of having 11 cohorts are that they get to know each other's intimacies: symptoms, deficits, aspirations and fears, and the benefits of a diversified group of people representing different cultures, personalities, lifestyles, life experiences, ages and professional callings. I have little family support due to conflict a great number of years ago.

My support group is much smaller. I have Jay, who is my PA (Personal Assistant) and dear lifelong friend, coming for five or six days a week for quite a number of hours both as a friend and worker. My father, who lives out-of-state, comes for long periodic sprints of time and talks daily on the phone and sometimes several times a day. I also have my Aunt, who is also my Godmother in Kentucky, who raises my spiritual being daily by phone with her love and wisdom. I also have a close sister (one of five siblings). I have a substantial loss of a second tier of friends whom I have lost along the way, which is typical for TBI survivors. I greatly value the few who have stayed. I also isolate myself rather than sharing my experience, for which I feel shame. This is especially due to my speech. I live independently with my service dog, who is my soulmate. I was very independent prior to my accident. I have the support of my rehabilitation team of therapists, doctors and my mentor Rick, all of whom I see frequently. Post-accident, Claudia and I have both become dependent.

While Claudia attends HTP, she also lives independently during the week. She lives in one place during the week and another on the weekends, including visits to home. Claudia's memory is different from mine. Having to move so frequently, she wakes up sometimes with confusion. Claudia can't remember where she is, for which she writes herself notes. She gets lost in her apartment and can't find the light switches or the phone. She gets lost in the neighborhood and in her grocery store. I live in the same house I have lived in since before my children were born, so I know it well. I have assistance during the weekdays in which I have someone take me to do errands or to do the shopping for me. I wake up in confusion in the middle of the night but for a very different reason. I have nightmares and flashbacks from my car crashes. Claudia does not remember her accident, so she has nothing to flashback to. Claudia and I both have adynamia, a neurologically based lack of vigor, spontaneity or animation. Claudia struggles with this to a greater extent than I do. Claudia and her cohorts do videotaping exercises to see how they appear to the world. I do voice recordings to see how I sound to the world while trying to break out of my speech difficulty, slow rate and monotone voice.

Claudia and I both have to learn to speak in full sentences with enough information to make sense and to elaborate. Claudia, like me, also works with a merciless effort to learn and then use compensatory strategies. Claudia wants to hide her newfound tools from her friends, even though they help her live her life (i.e., Post-It notes, notebooks, name cheat sheets). She does not want them to know she needs to rely on them, hence knowing she has a memory problem. In contrast, I am working on integrating my tools and strategies into everyday life, memory permitting. So, my tools are out in the open. Further, Claudia realizes she is not on autopilot anymore. What a great word! This is the reality of having a brain injury. We have to think about every single step in order to accomplish each individual task each and every time.

Commonalities

Among our similar attitudes, Claudia and I both are headstrong in that we are going to get back to work immediately following our program. We firmly believe this no matter what anyone has to say. We remain confident in our programs and ability to be successful, although no one has told either of us that we can get back to our previous selves. It is our assumption. From my journal:

I look realistically. in a fog – absent of mind struggling to end of day – mainly live in the monument – start all over very next day. my enduring – dissertation work trying to learn write a sentence – somehow been – for once write good sentence will be cured. more long-range thought of. she is gaining more knowledge wellness

Later that day, I wrote:

missing or not connecting in her head so productive her previous world/knowledge back – frustrating battle – wonder if ever. I need to win my battle.

I was trying to write that with hard work we will get through this and back to our stations in life.

In Claudia's early days of attending her rehabilitation program, another client tells her she will not work again as a doctor. This is appalling to me. I never even thought of that as a possibility. Claudia brushes it off as incongruent, and so do I. She thinks to herself that she is there to get better and back to work, which for her is seeing patients and teaching other doctors. I have full confidence that she will make it, and so will I – earning my doctorate and again seeing my clients/patients.

Claudia and I are akin as we share a high work ethic. As well we tend to border on the side of perfectionism. We are both involved in helping people, which entails numerous committees and meetings with busy work schedules. Hers are mainly inside the hospital, and mine are outside in the community. We value our determination, resilience and strong faith. Our analytical minds are of great importance. Independence, we both cherish. Then BANG!! She is crashed into by a car while riding her bicycle. My car is crashed into up to the front seat by a truck. Both our lives change significantly in that instant. Neither of us realize this until quite some time later. All that we value is no longer available to us.

My abilities, inner resources and values have been stolen! And I don't know how to articulate it. Similar to Claudia, who now knows how to express her new TBI cultural way of being, "We are different, we know it, and we would give much to have the dimensions of that loss understood, and thereby bridge the chasm between those of you who have not had this experience and those of us who have" (Osborn, 1998, p. XII). We both have significant memory loss, although Claudia's is even more severe than mine. She pleads that although others have moments of temporary forgetfulness, it does not cause a loss of their personhood, interests, profession and community service, as it has ours. Neither our work nor ourselves are familiar to us anymore.

I feel strange. My awareness is heightened by the many similarities I find with Claudia from early on in the book. Causing confusion, I have to check my reality. In my journal, I write:

> *Mind blowing – long to write – had to – hard to describe – I'm not sure, feeling same? fuzzy? – of déjà vu? – not quite – of looking in mirror? each new similar – felt strange – new similarity – the head, headaches – sleeping, but memory can't remember from beginning. Not using her right shoulder – unknown reason – maybe in rotator cuff me rotator – right – torn. startling when hear garden and roses – threw me for – expect similarities – can't explain. Felt visceral level and like this can't –. too similarities too soon in book. – very confused. How can this – hit too close to home. can 2 stories very differ degrees all kinds coping and not. same pieces. can't figure. Trying add more paragraphs not getting anywhere – sort this out – reading back. have 1 million typos – good metaphor happening for right now.* (I cleaned up the typos here for readability.)

In retrospect, I can decipher the sentiment into one sentence (which I did several years later on 10–18–15): *This is like someone writing what is in my head, tapping into my imprisoned thoughts, reading my mind that I cannot free.* The gist of my journal entry is how surreal it is to read so many similarities. I have not met another with TBI, but I know it is unique to each individual. No two are the same. In the beginning, as I reread, I find that Claudia has: her brain injury; headaches; sleeps a great deal of time initially; hurt her head, neck and right shoulder; a severe memory problem; audio and visual sensory overload with people and noise coming at her at the same time; and incredulously, her physical release is working in her garden with roses. My passion is working in my rose garden. On a visceral level, I feel confused and like this cannot be true. There are so many similarities so soon in the book. I wonder how two stories with many different degrees can have so many similarities. I find myself stuck in this reflection. I am also not aware yet of all the symptoms, so I do not realize our many differences at this time.

From the journal quote, in retrospect, I know that Claudia and I are both trying to get back to our doctoral work. Claudia finds solace puttering in her garden with roses. My solace is in my rose garden of many years that I find I can no longer tend. This is due to my right shoulder, neck and arm still out of commission and in great pain from the car crash and surgeries. I have the rose beds

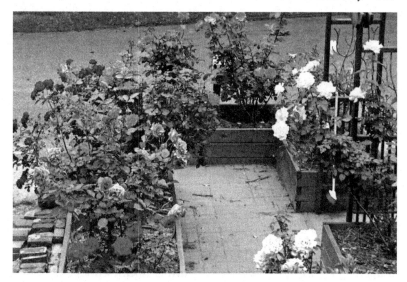

Figure 10.2 Dee's Healing Rose Garden

raised three feet with cedarwood and pavers through the middle in order to reach them, mainly with my left arm. I am filling my mind, body and spirit through the tantalizing inhalation of each distinctive scent. The vision of the delicate and blushing substantial blooms as well as vivid beauties (I have astonishing colors) and the prickly foreboding thorns to protect them have become my healing garden. My hand goes into the cool-ish earth under the nestled cedar mulch around each rose bush. I soak up the sun beating down on my long, open-back dress and a breeze blows gently, brushing my arms whisking my hair off of my face. I stretch forward a bit in my wheelchair to reach for the water jug. It is the fourth element of nature for me and my twelve American Beauty rose bushes in this healing garden. I have the earth, wind, sun and water. Feeling the spirit of tranquility years before, which I can recall when I am out here, I penned the following verses:

The Spirit of Tranquility

You search to beckon your senses of tranquility,
    to unlock your internal treasures,
and though this wealth may be exposed, the spiritual
    key must be discovered:

Allow yourself to recapture a precious moment,
   to rekindle that joyful feeling,
to re-view that wondrous, magical scene through
   the windows into your mind;

To actually hear the lulled tones of quiescence,
   to inhale the fragrance of your thought,
to allow the serenity buried within you to
   flow and calm at will.

(Genetti, 1992)

My precious moments are in my rose garden. I am quite amazed that Claudia and I share this same passion and are able to find physical release working with roses.

Claudia and I also have flooding thoughts, an organic problem caused by the brain injury. She describes her thinking as becoming confusing, ineffectual and painfully slow. Further, she describes that trying to hear another person's words is like listening to a symphony with cotton plugging her ears. This correlates with my flooding thoughts, which to me sound like static, like someone turning the radio stations fast with the volume on full blast and not settling on a single station. It causes swift, incomprehensible emotional reactions. From Claudia, "my mental switchboard is awash in strong emotions even though, at the time, I am unaware of any emotion" (Osborn, 1998, p. 62).

My rage, which I cannot understand, is also shared by Claudia. There is a visceral connection between us as she describes running after a taxi driver yelling obscenities. She admits knowing her explosive rage was not proportional to the offense she felt. "I was still seething long after the taillights had vanished in the afternoon gloom. . . . As my rage faded, I felt embarrassed and dismayed. . . . Behavior like this was so out of character for me." (Osborn, 1998, p. 177). It is out of character for me, as well. Rage is a behavioral change of the TBI sequelae. It is disinhibited, quick and uncontrollably blurts out. After an angry outburst of rage from me, I wrote in my journal:

> *Every little change takes a monument this effort for me to switch
> my brain around – angry outbursts if and when I have to let go of
> memory in retrain for change – to think differently – the change –
> my mind is fixated and settled before the obstacle trying to hold
> tight – fall apart – angry outbursts if and when I have to let go
> memory for the change – frustrating – instant emotion out-pour –
> rage. But me unaware emotions.*

Before now, I always had irreprehensible self-control.

Fatigue is another commonality, although I think mine is more pronounced. Claudia tries a job trial at the hospital where she does medical secretary work in Admissions for two hours in the morning and two hours in the afternoon. She fatigues tremendously and zones out during her lunch break. She cannot wait to get home and get to bed due to exhaustion. Then, she starts again the next day. Claudia's schedule, too, is governed by her new TBI cultural characteristics. In this case, it is persistent fatigue. Proving to be too much cognitively, her workload in the afternoon is redirected to caring for the garden in the atrium for two hours. Misting the plants is physical rather than mental work and far less fatiguing. Dr. Claudia Osborn is trained by a high school student in how to mist plants, which is astounding to me but gratifying to Claudia at her new level of functioning. The gardening works out, but the morning job does not. Claudia's memory gets in the way of her responsibilities. It is over her head. Claudia graduates from HTP, and the work trial ends. Claudia's day program at HTP has been18 months. My road through this period has been very slow but steadier.

11 Road to Recovery
Beginning of Re-identification

A Fellow Traveler

I have really met a fellow traveler with TBI through Dr. Claudia Osborn's book. I am developing a relationship with Claudia and responding emotionally as her story unfolds. As I read the book, I realize this is my first peer with whom I am sharing that I have a TBI. I feel I am becoming emotionally attached to her recovery. I am getting to know Claudia as a person who really is a fellow traveler. Looking at my journey, I wonder if it may map onto hers. I am hoping to take strength from some of her successes. I relate with Claudia in cultural terms of new values, beliefs, attitudes and experiences. It is gratifying and relieving to hear Claudia articulate my daily thoughts, concerns and happenings. It is also reassuring to hear the not-so-great symptomatology, an affirmation of the totality of the symptoms my doctor has acknowledged in me. Somebody else knows my pain and suffering. She understands my fervent hope and adamant position that I will be back to my doctoral studies and trauma clients. As Claudia fights willfully to get back to doctoring, I believe in her tenacity and hard work. I believe that the undertaking of this awe-inspiring book will unquestionably conclude with her comeback to her "old" life. I share the acknowledgment that it will be very hard work, although I do not understand what this will entail.

I quoted Claudia in a note I put in my journal:

> *As soon as I reached home, I sat with my notebook and tried to organize my thoughts. I prayed I had communicated some of my litany. Please fix my thinking and reasoning, coach. Repair my memory. Make me a doctor again. Just get me to my job on time.*
>
> (Osborn, 1998, p. 77)

DOI: 10.4324/9781003428510-15

I had to listen twice to these statements. It could have almost been written by me, as I write notes on my computer when I get home from seeing Rick. The clue is that it is written in complete sentences with clear thoughts, but my thoughts are in my head, too. Claudia and I share a parallel sentiment of urgency to get fixed and get back to our old lives, our stations in life. As well we hope that we get enough information out of our brains to make sense.

To my shock and dismay, a not-so-good part of the TBI cultural road we travel is the word *permanent*. Claudia claims this word stripped her of hope and shattered her dreams. Claudia wonders, as do I, how she can continue to exist as an unrecognizable, undesirable being living with a deficient brain. Bearable was her/our fated brain injuries because they are temporary. "Permanent injury meant I had already lost. My job. My identity. My life" (Osborn, 1998, p. 116). Claudia found out, to her horror, that everyone at the HTP program had lost his or her old self. "Forever, as in permanent injury, *permanent!*" (Osborn, 1998, p. 116). She feels numb about her self-knowledge and cannot turn back the clock to when she unknowingly believed her losses were all fixable. She acknowledges having a long way to go to reach emotional acceptance of her head injury persona. I am speechless and breathless . . . and then I fall asleep.

Depression overcomes Claudia, "The one feeling that was readily identifiable was the consuming depression that followed each jolt of memory about the permanence of my injuries. The trigger was invariably related to my desire to do medicine" (Osborn, 1998, p. 126). Of her rehab, Claudia wrote, "I thought rehabilitation meant **a path** to take me home, to resume my former life, to return to the person I think of as me" (Osborn, 1998, p. 133). Claudia thinks it will be impossible to sort her feelings while trying to write her third short speech for HTP. She does not think it possible to put words to her questions regarding her future and what she has been through.

Claudia wonders, "What was it I had to accept? What were my abilities and potential?" (Osborn, 1998, p. 186). She has also written, "When I saw the words on the page, I realized they weren't about me. They were about a person I would never be again" (Osborn, 1998, p. 178). And a bit further, "I was disgusted with the worthless person I had become." When I hear these words on these pages, I feel mirror image feelings that I, too, will be deprived of myself. It is astonishing to find someone who can articulate my dreadful thoughts, emotions and suffering – exactly. I am with her. I have helped many others articulate their emotions, especially with my words in my poetry book (Genetti, 1992), and here Claudia has put words to mine unspoken. As I am losing hope for myself, I am grateful for her transparency, but I hold on even tighter to my belief that Claudia will absolutely get back to doctoring. I feel my life depends on it. I think, why else would she write this book if not to show her triumph?

Claudia is told she has to find a new purpose. Presented matter-of-factly, the topic seemed subtle. It was devastating to me, though. There was a clear assumption that things about Claudia/about me will not change back, a continuous message in various ways throughout our rehabilitation programs. Claudia is told, "We can't put your brain in a cast and mend it like a broken leg," and "Strategies don't cure problems, they ameliorate them" (p. 116). Claudia stated for both of us, "When I said 'better,' I meant all better" (p. 116). Those phrases registered for the first time to Claudia, and I unnervingly took notice. Claudia is told that no one can predict just how far she can go in her recovery, that she should have hope to strive as far as she can, but to know there is a ceiling. She is told emphatically, "You won't get everything back" (p. 119). I am told this one month in the future from when I finish the book. I adamantly refuse to believe she will not make it.

More cultural discoveries are that the second cycle of Claudia's rehabilitation program is to increase and master strategies and gain emotional and intellectual acceptance of her/our new selves. Wow! I am just barely out of denial. Claudia's adjustment is not yet there. She is told, "You continue to measure your performance against your pre-injury standards. . . . You are asking too much of yourself. You are engaging in what is called maximalist thinking" (p. 168). Claudia discovers her cohorts have all suffered the loss of old friends and finds that they all polish their use of props which include daily timers and alarms, tape cassettes, lists and notebooks to name a few. I use many of the same. Claudia's essential way of functioning is her memory and organizer notebook.

"I tried desperately to hold onto my thoughts, to decide what to do and then to act on that decision" (p. 62), Claudia exclaims. My thoughts strive for the same, but they are seldom carried out that way. Claudia and her cohorts at HTP mirror my predicaments, but I understand more easily the experiences they describe. Of my own experiences, I cannot make sense. I do not hold the insight or imagination to see myself, as I describe in my journal, not being able to cope with and heal my trauma-therapist self. After hearing my notes several times, I realize these are familiar words to Claudia that mimic my thoughts and frustrated reality, which I feel prolong my recovery.

Claudia makes attempts at work in several ways. First, she writes a medical report for a lecture at HTP. She feels successful in her research and other efforts but claims it comes at a price. She spent two weeks preparing what should have taken one hour to execute. She wonders how she can keep up that level of effort. She also wonders if this were a real teaching situation how she can prepare the material on time. Her conclusion is, "But it tells me teaching medicine would be a problem. The lecture stuff I knew. Medicine changes constantly. I would have to learn new material in order to teach it and I was concerned by these implications in terms of a future vocation" (Osborn, 1998, p. 177). Her future vocation back to doctoring and teaching medicine does not happen. I am crushed! I have to reconsider my own aspirations or face a different reality for the first time – overwhelming.

Our paths divert when Claudia does not return to her profession because, at this point, I am still adamantly trying to return to mine. It has unexpectedly become a vehicle for my own post-traumatic growth to now have to forge a path without Claudia. She has been my guide for an important period of time.

Analysis, Interpretation and Re-identification

Over My Head (Osborn, 1998) and Dr. Claudia Osborn is a paradigm for my early recovery. Reading the book has been effectual. I have learned some of the treatments for TBI. I have learned I am not all alone with the many symptoms I struggle with daily and how they go together. I relate to Claudia even though we have many differences in our TBI presentations. She is a doctor who wants to get back to medicine, which is a difficult thing to do. I relate to her new cultural values, beliefs, attitudes and not-always-politically correct behaviors, such as rage. I am now forced to face my own recovery and reality, which Claudia has done with the survivor group at HTP and a new lifestyle. I have relearned skills for reading, comprehension, writing and note-taking.

Claudia and I both wanted a role model to be able to know what we were up against with brain injuries. We wanted to know how long and what it would take to heal so we could get on with life. That is not possible as every brain injury, hence recovery, is unique. No two are the same. From my journal:

> *Acceptance of limitations could be less emotional if clearly defined.*
> *I would like to know what has happened to me? What is TBI? What*
> *is PTSD? What is MDD, even though I know some of the answers as*

a therapist it is totally different when personal, and what are the limits or more importantly what are the goals probable for me to reach? If I, or Claudia only knew what the whole deficit entails – what is the deal here? we could deal with in a much better way. be more accepting understand Claudia well. Grasp the specifics of her limitations – I could move on faster and less emotional if I knew the same – what I am up against and then working to overcome what I can and relearn or drop the things not possible/probable – maybe until I was the best I could possibly be.

In contemplation, I became aware of what it feels like to have a TBI through Claudia and her cohorts. They have been role models for me. I discovered that recovery from TBI is not about returning 100% to your old self but rather finding as much of your old self as is intact and finding/building a new identity, changing your perspective, and learning how to live it. I was border crossing into unfamiliar territory with encounters of others of difference who became others of similarity. They, too, voiced their dismay about a life not their own and were lost after TBI, having to find a new identity. In me, I discovered a non-competent person trying to perform my life and not doing it very well.

In this new culture of TBI, due to disability impairment on different levels, Claudia and I have a change in our beliefs and attitudes. We both believe we will break out of the stigmatizing culture through hard work and diligence, even when we are told it is permanent and that room for recovery is possible, but there is a ceiling, albeit an unknown ceiling. We both wonder if life happiness is possible after TBI. Claudia and I agree in our beliefs that people, friends and family members can no longer depend on us, the very people who lean on us, due to our impairments. We believe there are negative implications for our future vocations, which Claudia has reckoned with, but I have not. Losing our identity and having to create a new one is paramount. Claudia comes to believe that building a new life can be delightful, whereas I am trying to cling to my old one. Memories of my old life have faded dramatically, and my emotional stronghold is lessening. I come to believe eventually, as Claudia does, that we must rebuild a new identity or wither and die.

We both have a new cultural attitude about redefining what "successful" now means. The concern is about future vocation. What will that look like, and do we have or can we obtain the skills? Claudia and I both express a need for a vision of an achievable future in this new culture. Our families are both confident in our ability to overcome adversity. But we are not because this is a new and very challenging identity. We believe that becoming a member of this culture is not just an adversity. Claudia communicates that she feels "less than." She wants to hide her new tools such as Post-It notes, timer and notebook to remind her of necessary people, places and things. Her attitude is to hide her impairments from friends. She and I both feel the essence of stigma, including through the loss of friends. I do not go out of my way to hide in this new culture, though. "I was not this damaged shell of a person. I couldn't be. I remembered and loved the person I was. That was the real me" (Osborn, 1998, p. 118). This is my sentiment exactly – exactly! I cannot say it any better. In my journal, I had written previously to reading:

> *I am still a shell of what I used to be even though I gained back a lot. I had only up to go. I can't hold a candle to the original me before the accident.*

We both can now have pride in our accomplishments, especially when they take an extraordinary amount of time to achieve. An anecdote, for example, is when Claudia got a library card and took out a book all by herself, which took three hours. I felt swollen with pride for her. She was wondering who she could tell that would get the depth and gravity with which the feat took. She did not allow her usual feeling of embarrassment to take over. She instead had pride. I share that great pride when accomplishing what seems to others as a tiny independent act. Claudia is settling into her new identity while I am starting to relate to others again. This is an important step for me since I withdrew from most of my relationships. I also found that Claudia is trying to journal her experience and also writes cryptically. She, too, does not always understand what she is trying to document for her memories.

Claudia finds she cannot do her previous job as a medical doctor nor teach the interns. She does not have the skills anymore, she found through her exercises at HTP. From my journal:

> *Claudia finding out she cannot do her job anymore gave me more determination to get back to my doctoral program and finish my dissertation, but unfortunately it does not give me the skills. When someone tells me I cannot do a thing, if it is worth doing, I try twice as hard to do it and in half the time it would take another person. Tough ramifications for myself.*

The next day, from my reflection journal:

> *I had depression due to the loss of me. Different from Claudia, I had suicidal ideation so strong and unrelenting since this second car crash. It haunts me or shadows, feels ingrained deeply and I can't put many words to it. The idea that Claudia may not get back to being a doctor still devastates me and gives me less hope.*

My depression worsens to Major Depressive Disorder. I continue to see my trauma therapist for EMDR and other modalities, including talk therapy. Flashbacks and PTSD symptoms overwhelm me daily. Through learning to read and write with *Over My Head* (Osborn, 1998), I become more educated with the complications and the sequelae of TBI. A lot of the sequelae are co-occurring with my PTSD symptomatology. Flashbacks, hypervigilance and hyper startle response are triggered by the loud noise of cars and trucks rushing by on the Route 93 traffic way behind and below my house. The noise triggers soon transfer to other loud noises inside my house. This is a part of my hell that Claudia did not have to experience.

From my journal:

> *I am almost at the end of her journey and Claudia says she has come to grips with this life. She imparts that she is ready to move on and claim this new life with hope, feeling pleasure, and happily looking forward. Even though she is happy, I am unhappy with her results. Do I have a right to feel this way? I expected that after going to a second session at the Head Trauma Program she would have enough tools to get back to doctoring at some level. I feel angry, like she was short changed after all that rehab. Claudia seemed too accepting and to embrace suddenly her new life. I wanted to hear more of what she went through at the turning point. I suppose she was bearing the intolerable, but I thought she was still fighting that. As a therapist I did not hear the struggle before the supposed acceptance of "pleasurable." I want more for her. I want Claudia to be able to read and write and improve to regain more tools for her memory problems. I want her to be able to live in a society she once enjoyed.*

I realize now I want *me* to live in the society *I* once enjoyed.

In another journal reflection, I wrote:

> *I feel that Claudia suddenly accepted her fate that she calls new life, without looking back. I am not able to do that and do not know how*

a driven woman with all her talents would be able to either. At least tell me how! I caught her frustration, but not the bridge that helped her acceptance, which also takes confidence or maybe withdrawal. Is that the bargaining phase? I don't know. Something is missing before acceptance. I felt angry that she did not seem to look back during graduation time, a time for reflection on your accomplishments and deficits, a time for thinking now versus then, and what has been in the middle, and then finally letting go of some past and looking realistically at the future. I hope for her. I fear for me.

Claudia states at the end of her book, "I was a happy woman before my injury, I am a happy one today" (p. 232). My reflection journal:

I am devastated. I presume that if you want to lead your life instead of wallowing, you have to come to terms with it. I do not think I can drop or change my life to embrace another, not again. I have been there, done that after my first car crash. It took lots and lots of energy, courage, soul-searching, letting go and rebuilding to make my life worthwhile. I do not believe I have it in me again. I work hard to recover. It is exhausting. Now I am trying to find where I fit and find what I have to use or give. I also was a happy woman before and am trying to be a happier one now. For me it is not working.

Looking toward the greater social context, as I try to piece myself back together, I am met with discrimination because of the brain injury. Unfortunately, this includes discrimination by others with disabilities, even though I was accepted with my paraplegia by many. The disability rights movement worked in a second phase to create a disability culture of collective identity, with cross-disabilities to include all disabilities. Unfortunately, stigma still abounds, especially with non-physical disabilities.

I full-heartedly believed Claudia would be back in her field in some capacity. I did not want her to be happy with this new life. I lost hope in my own recovery. In my devastation, I reached out and wrote to Claudia. She wrote back and encouraged me to keep going. She imparted that the most important aspect of her recovery was her life coach or mentor, as I told her about Rick. Claudia urged me to continue my path with Rick. With time passed and her book published, which took ten years to write, Claudia told me she has a full life with love shared with her partner and is now doing motivational speaking. She has also recently begun teaching a first-year medical program at a university. I am happy for and proud of her. I am full of ambivalence for me.

12 Taking a Toll Road
Concurrent Mental Health Issues

During the second half of this third and fourth year post-TBI, my mental health is taking a deep turn for the worse. *A pivotal moment:* my depression deteriorates to an even lower level. On January 8, 2009, my one sister with whom I am closest dies suddenly at age 48. Deb beat breast cancer, but at this time, several years later, it metastasized. She developed complications and died within a very short period. It is hitting me harshly. We spoke daily for most of an hour. Sharing a close relationship, we also shared the same sense of humor and writing of poetry. Another piece of me is gone with her loss. From the limited socializing that I hold onto, I now withdraw further.

However, a small miracle comes about in her death. During Debbie's last days, I, along with many of the estranged family members on one side, hold a vigil around her. This is for support in her special hospital room, where she is receiving comfort and care in order to pass in peace. Renewed relationships are bonding, including with me. This is a wish that Debbie has had for a very long time. It is unfortunate it is in her death that we are able to bring about her united family wish. Consoling one another, I relate to others as I accept needing others for support. As well, I am giving from my heart at this time. My TBI sequelae, especially my speech, visibly shakes everyone uncomfortably during these days and nights we are together. As I reflect, I realize that I had not processed my profound losses and predicament until after Deb's sudden death. I had not been able to critically reflect. Critical reflection is problematic in the darkness of PTSD and TBI.

Neuropsychological Evaluation

In March 2009, it becomes obvious that I have great impenetrability in making enough gains in my work and my writing despite a mammoth effort. I am stalled. I am stuck. Losing steam, Rick suggests I see

DOI: 10.4324/9781003428510-16

Dr. Chi, my physiatrist, for physical medicine and a charge person for my brain injury. In turn, he, along with Dr. Bob, my PCP with whom I have a collaborative relationship, refers me to Dr. Jacob, a neuropsychologist. It is determined that a neuropsychological assessment is the only way to formally assess brain function to see where I am.

In April 2009, I am given a series of tests over three different days with several days of breaks in between. This is due to the doctor's feeling that my fatigue sets in, and I glaze over. Dr. Jacob reports that he stopped the testing "due to extreme fatigue, which would not allow her to continue at her brightest. Word retrieval and intellectual stamina were the biggest impediments." Traditionally, the test is administered in one day, sometimes two.

Along with my history of the motor vehicle crash with brief loss of consciousness and mild traumatic brain injury, Dr. Jacob reports in April 2009 that I:

> Present with severe cognitive impairments that are of sufficient magnitude to warrant concern about her safety to perform household activities (e.g., cooking), and have dramatically decreased functional status.

I had flunked cooking on the stove and microwave after three occupational therapy sessions. I was told I was not safe to cook. I was given the solution of heating up frozen dinners in the microwave, which caused a quandary. I do not like frozen dinners as they contain far too much sodium. I previously loved to cook, making home-cooked food daily. I do have others who occasionally bring me a dish, and at times, I cook with supervision, which takes an astronomical amount of time. For now, though, I am primarily stuck with buying pre-made dinners from my grocery store bakery area. I have difficulty and need help for performing these and other previously simple household activities. It is frustrating that I am still so dependent in these third and fourth years post-TBI. Other cognitive results by Dr. Jacob were significant for:

> 1) Profound impairment of attentional function, with rapid cognitive fatigue, distractibility, and severe impairment of sustained and selective attention. 2) Variability across tasks of executive functioning with intact novel reasoning ability, but severe impairment of timed thought generation, cognitive flexibility, as well as some evidence of perseveration and stimulus bound behavior on tasks of rudimentary motor control. 3) Language impairments

with reduced verbal fluency, word-retrieval deficits, and difficulty with high-level language organization and verbal expression. 4) Impairment of visual constructional ability. 5) A severe attentionally based memory impairment with reduced acquisition and retrieval of information, and poor performance on recognition tasks. 6) Motor symptoms consistent with impersistence during complex tasks (e.g., writing) such that she can write several words accurately, but slows with repeated trials and eventually stops completely unable to continue. Beyond the cognitive assessment, from a psychological perspective Ms. Genetti is also currently struggling with symptoms of depression and PTSD related to her multiple traumas.

Additionally, Dr. Jacob reports that very likely contributing to my reduced cognitive efficiency at this time are:

re-experiencing of trauma, PTSD and depression, as well as the effects of ongoing pain (related to physical injuries) and poor sleep maintenance (secondary to sleep apnea, ongoing pain and PTSD reactions).

Further, Dr. Jacob references one of the referral questions regarding the potential of my return to graduate school. He communicates that:

At the current time, it is extremely difficult to imagine that she would be able to handle these tasks. Her decreased attention capacity, rapid fatigue, reduced memory, and overall level of behavioral disorganization are of sufficient magnitude that they are resulting in impairments of independent activities of daily living, which are far less demanding than the rigors of data analysis and academic writing. Unless there is significant improvement in her cognitive status and endurance, it is also extremely difficult to imagine her participation in continued professional activities.

Moreover, regarding potential cognitive recommendations, Dr. Jacob recognizes that I have been working extensively with my speech therapist and with Atech. The focus has been on strategies to facilitate writing and provide assistance with specific phases of my project leading to my dissertation, using Dragon Naturally Speaking. Dr. Jacob adds that my level of difficulty with memory and organizing my thoughts is combined with issues of difficulty with physical writing. He recommends even greater emphasis on a computer with speech recognition, which I have. In fact, Dr. Jacob reports that he would like me to have a laptop mounted on my wheelchair. Sitting on my lap throughout the day became the stratagem to compensate in order to fulfill Dr. Jacob's recommendation that "as much as possible in order to make notes, and facilitate with day-to-day activities such as dictating grocery lists or ideas as they come to her." Putting this into practice proved to be *im*practical, though we try to keep it as near me as possible. Likewise, Dr. Jacob recommends I continue with all my therapies for the integration of compensatory strategies regarding activities of daily living.

Shockingly, my traditionally high IQ tested as borderline intelligence. This is distressing as it certainly does not project the needs and ability to learn scholarly writing and finish my dissertation. This news is shaming on one hand and non-comprehensible on the other.

Continued Psychotherapy

I continue in counseling that began in December of 2007. It had taken some time to find, but I was finally referred to a trauma therapist, Ellie, through a colleague. Initially seeking EMDR to address symptoms of PTSD, it soon became obvious that I first needed help in far more basic ways. I felt totally disoriented. My experience was fragmented and incomprehensible to me. Ellie's clinical note shows:

> Dee had very little support and felt helpless and dependent for the first time in her memory. She found herself unable to cope with even simple tasks, such as making a grocery list or remembering to eat. She had not processed the traumatic automobile crash that led to her current symptoms and triggered the re-experiencing of the car crash that left her paraplegic years before, and other traumatic events. The traumatic reliving of these events left her feeling terrified much of the time.

Ellie also reports observing my expression of intense frustration at my impaired ability to function cognitively due to the impact of my TBI. We quickly shifted from EMDR to address my PTSD with talk therapy and TAPPAS, as I could not follow the EMDR protocol cognitively. I talk about both accidents, the impact of the second accident on my life and other traumatic events from my past that have all come crashing down and out at this time. I thought I had dealt with all my fodder. For many years, I had no symptoms until this second accident. I felt healed. As I progressed sometime later, EMDR did indeed help my recovery.

Ellie questions me as to what motivates me in the face of another catastrophic loss, as well as great emotional and physical suffering. She records that I speak frequently about my speech language therapy and my intent on returning to writing my doctoral dissertation. Ellie also records that I have done extensive preparation and research for my dissertation. During this timeframe, Ellie's observations in a note to my doctor reveal:

> Dee has significant cognitive impairment along with significantly impaired short-term memory in sessions. She shows evidence of being tangential, though she is usually able to identify it and return to the intended focus. Dee gets frustrated when unable to say something because she is overwhelmed by many thoughts at once, and could not hold on to any of them. Difficulty with word finding proceeded. Dee could only grasp one small concept at a time and would end up "spaced out" when presented with multiple or complex ideas. She demonstrated difficulty making lists of what she needed to do, and reported that she was unable to follow through on identified tasks, getting confused by the necessary steps or frustrated and overwhelmed when things did not go as she had planned.

Many of our sessions are spent trying to help me make lists of things I need to do. As well we are problem-solving, processing incidents that make me feel helpless and angry and strategizing how to manage such situations that I have difficulty enumerating. I reveal the intense shame I feel about my diminished cognitive functioning and consequent unwillingness to contact my friends. This furthers my isolation. Ellie elaborates in a note that I demonstrate the characteristic profile of brain injury, which leads to disruptions in intellect, emotionality and control of behavior. She writes that it is difficult for me to hold onto the whole big picture of my troubles.

Ellie reveals my disorganized status and inability to prioritize in a note on 10–8–09:

> Dee had no preference for one food or blouse over another, and no task took precedence over another in her mind, to order a delivery of oil or fold the laundry.

Further, she reports:

> Dee could not organize her thoughts, her home was disorga-
> nized for the first time in her life, and she was unable to put
> things away where they belonged. Dee showed utter exhaustion
> at the end of a session and stated as much for other appoint-
> ments. Even simple tasks, such as paying bills or writing an
> e-mail were overwhelming and led to procrastination or intense
> and protracted effort and extreme frustration. Dee has shown
> extraordinary resiliency throughout her life, but feels she is
> 'losing that battle,' feeling that she overcame overwhelming
> challenges before . . . "I'm not 'me' anymore. More and more
> of me is slipping away every day. I can't find 'me.'" Dee has a
> loss of ability to trust.

At this time, I disclose to Ellie that I have lost touch with what it
means to engage in everyday activities, that I don't know how to
get back and that everything terrifies me. Unresolved issues from
the past are recycling with a vengeance. Eroded by the intensity of
my pain and loss are my defense mechanisms. I am in the throes of
extreme grief, and my emotional resources are inadequate. Trying
to cope, I wrote in my journal:

> *Trying to think I beat odds before so I will get back, but I don't
> think I believe myself anymore.*

Another observation notates Ellie:

> Her very painful shoulder/rotator cuff, neck and pectoral mus-
> cles injury from the second car accident makes it impossible for
> her to function as independently as she had.

My physicality is problematic. My debilitating injury results in two
surgeries, a number of cortisone injections – two under fluoroscopy,
trigger point injections and acupuncture. I also undergo physical
therapy involving stretching exercises and massage, ultrasound, a
TNS unit for pain management and the use of an at-home dynasplint
shoulder positioning apparatus. My arm, dangling from my shoulder
in pain, is difficult to move in most upward and outward motions.
My pectoral muscle is in spasms, pulling my underarm to my chest.
My neck, with nerve impingements, is also pulled downward due
to the pectoral muscle spasms. The whole region is inflamed. This

makes it difficult to do almost anything with my arm and hand that zing from nerve impingement. I transfer my body from my wheel-chair to the couch, bed or other chair by lifting myself with both arms and moving my body over, then grabbing each leg and pulling them over with me. I can no longer lift myself with my right arm hence transfers are very challenging.

Ellie quotes from me in her notes, "Instead of 4 limbs I only have the use of one now, my left arm." And further notes:

> This physical limitation contributed to a loss of autonomy and feelings of extreme vulnerability. Dee described that as a result of the TBI she is no longer able to perform what would have been simple, routine tasks for her before the car crash. She states that the simplest task is a Herculean labor for her. She often found herself too daunted, disorganized or discouraged by tasks to complete them.

With observations of my downward spiraling, Ellie writes:

> In April of 2009, Dee underwent extensive neuropsychologi-cal testing, which posited a poor prognosis for her recovery at the level of function needed to complete her doctoral disserta-tion. She had been confident that she would recover soon, write her dissertation and continue with her plans to open a trauma clinic for women victims/survivors of domestic violence and their children. Dee was devastated by the report. Observing this devastation was evident in the hopelessness and desperation she manifested in her sessions.

And with thoughts of my sister Deb's upcoming one-year anniver-sary of her death, Ellie's clinical note reveals:

> The one sister with whom Dee had the most loving and healthy relationship with had a sudden exacerbation of her cancer and died unexpectedly within two months. The positive attitude Dee managed to sustain for the first two years appeared destroyed. She went into a profound depression. She was faced for the first time with the belief that she may not be able to transcend her brain injury as she had for other traumatic events in her life, that neither her extraordinary resiliency, her willingness to work hard, nor her tenacity would help her recover her previous level of cognitive function. And she lost one of her primary supports.

I am reminded of a poem I wrote in 1989 as I tried desperately to become able-bodied but realized it was not possible:

The Wrath of Death

I lay here consumed in total despair,
The black wrath of death is drawing me near.

The end is here, with a final letting go,
It's the only **end means** to this arduous tow.

I have no fear of death inside of me
'cause relief will kill the overwhelming anxiety.

No one can help me, though some people have tried.
I'm filled with empty hopes, and out and out lies.

My emotions have been tested – unwound them all,
Like unravelling yarn off a six year old ball.

They now are left hanging, all jumbled and intense.
I can't lock them up, 'till I can make sense.

They've tested and pushed to the very end of my strength
And they found I am only bound by one single length.

I've worked real hard, I've worked real strong
But all of my efforts have turned out wrong.

The single length of yarn, that is all that is left
Will be used up within days – my life will not be kept.

(Genetti, 1992)

As my depression deepens, Ellie observes episodes symptomatic of both TBI and PTSD. They are irritability and anger from the brain injury, which intensify into episodes of rage. At times, episodes are precipitated by flashbacks; at other times with seemingly no precipitants. Episodes are found both in sessions and by telephone. Quoted in Ellie's clinical notes:

"I have rage and I explode and I don't know what to do with it." Dee reported that she hated and was embarrassed by the outbursts, but also felt less powerlessness confronting people who were letting her down.

It is during this time period that I find out my health insurance is denying further coverage for my speech and language therapy, twice weekly, because I am making progress too slowly. I firmly know this therapy organizes my life. It helps me to think and understand and is my primary hope for returning to optimal cognitive function. Out of sheer necessity, I manage to pay privately as my life literally depends on these sessions. As I divulged earlier, my sessions become once every two weeks and then three weeks for financial reasons, which is very disorganizing. I go from seeing Rick about eight times a month to two to three times a month. I feel increasingly depressed and hopeless.

13 Speed Bumps
Co-morbidity with TBI and PTSD

Depression

In trying to understand more about my symptoms and increased depression, I look toward the greater social context. This happens later when I am able to do research and write this book. A closer look at depression shows, as well as being a frequent symptom of PTSD, it is the single most common psychiatric disorder associated with TBI. I find that TBI symptoms and depression combine to construct a vicious cycle. Whereas depression increases TBI symptoms, TBI symptoms deepen depression. A contrasting view on depression questions whether a lack of awareness or insight is protective against depression with regard to the severity of the deficits of the individual with TBI. A third viewpoint found that more insight brings about depression. A fourth view found that an increase in one's understanding of their situation and cognitive abilities may help those with TBI cope better with difficulties facing them. I find through my research that in the first year post-injury, 20%–40% of TBI survivors suffer from depression. After the first year post-injury, the prevalence increases with time for those with depression.

Another significant emotional factor of TBI is the association with suicide risk, which touches my life in this timeframe. The estimated rates of suicidal ideation following TBI range from 22%–28%. In one study of individuals with a history of mild to severe TBI, 17.4% over a five year period reported suicide attempts, and most had no prior history of suicidal behavior. It is estimated TBI survivors are 1.55 to 3 times more likely to complete suicide than those in the general public who have not sustained a TBI. Suicidal feelings mixed with feelings from my first car crash after becoming paraplegic brought up poems of my earlier struggles:

DOI: 10.4324/9781003428510-17

Committed To A Living Death

In my deep and dark despair,
　I truly wish there were someone here,
To listen to me, might help me bear
　The despondent thoughts I've begun to fear.

Throughout the day, my thoughts I dread
　Of earnestly believing I'm better off dead.
To drown these thoughts swimming 'round my head,
　I long to close my eyes, and die in bed.

An abundant load of physical pain,
　I silently carry this tremendous strain.
My twisted body feels its energy drain;
　Anguish is flowing through every vein.

A burden I am to have to depend,
　Because I can't stand, or even bend.
The outside world, I cannot attend.
　My worth here on earth, I can't defend.

A commitment I made, my promise I keep.
　To not take this life, my words you do reap.
But confined in this body, I feel really deep,
　Is much more tormenting than forever sleep.
(Genetti, 1992)

Anxiety

I find I have a lot of unexpressed anger and anxiety in these third and fourth years. I feel complete horror and helplessness at having been injured so severely . . . again. My research shows that anxiety is a common contributing factor in the aftermath of suffering from a TBI and also PTSD. Having a plight of both anxiety and TBI, another vicious cycle is created. Resulting in a reduced capacity for memory and cognition, anxiety and stress weaken attention. Thereby, the more I feel anxious due to memory tribulations, the more likely my cognitive function will be worsened. Starting to feel anxious due to troubles with memory, anxiety will reign, making it more difficult for me to remember. Having even more memory troubles produces even more anxiety, and the cycle continues. Cataclysmic fear, anxiety and numbness experienced as a lack of meaning and emotional connection are core to post-traumatic stress characteristics in cases of brain injury. I am experiencing strongly. I am reconnecting with a poem I penned during flashbacks from my first car crash.

Anxiety

Consumed in hazy gloominess
Clouding every thought
A frenzy whirling inside me
Frantic and distraught.

Dazed with flooded thoughts and feelings
Flashing through my brain
Anxious to slow down the process
Before I go insane.

An explosion of emotions
Triggering in me
A volcanic eruption spewing –

Ashes I shall be.

(Genetti, 1992)

Flashbacks

I am suffering intrusive thoughts of my trauma, evident as nightmares, flashbacks, images, thoughts and feelings, which are constant. Feeling numb, or being numb, because there is no feeling connected with it and, due to my brain injury, my participation in significant activities has ended. I avoid people, places and activities associated with the trauma. I have a great loss of ability to trust.

In Figure 13.1, I made a visual depiction of my experiences with PTSD as the flashbacks zoomed in on me. Many were just as bits and pieces but in poetic verse. I overlaid them to show the flashing and astounding motion. The center picture, which accompanies the poem called *The Wheelman* literally portrays me embodying the wheelchair, as if the wheelchair was an appendage of my physical being.

Both car crashes occurred on the same highway, Route I-93, the dreadful highway where I was knocked off my trajectory not once but twice, just one mile apart. Both were caused by men who hit the car I was in, inflicting a violation on my person – one with his large

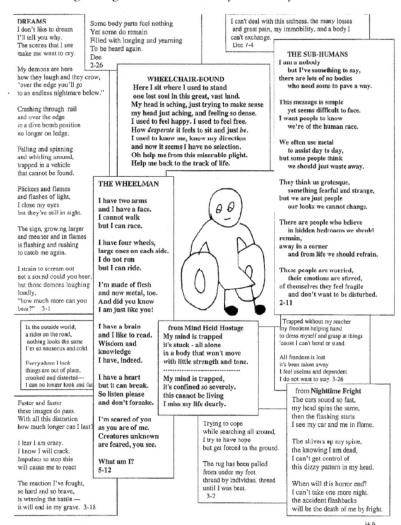

Figure 13.1 Flashbacks and Nightmares (Genetti, 1992)

truck and the other with his van. I experience these crashes as a violation of me, an infringement, destructive, damaging. Other similarities include they are both men who walked away from the crashes they caused, and both were driving a company vehicle, leading to lesser feelings of culpability. Both crashes happened on a clear and sunny morning. The first driver even had the exact same birthday as me, including my birth year. Route I-93 is also behind and below my backyard, so I hear it constantly. Both male drivers took from me my independence, power, control and sense of peace.

Out in my now narrowed world in an automobile, especially on the highway, I try to change my structures of meaning and expectation to diminish the heightened feelings, anxiety and nausea I have. My hope is that I can be a rider on the road again. I work assiduously to try to alter my immediate judgment and belief that a car is going to be my coffin. My view is slowly transforming, which has been just outside my awareness. It now can be heard if I listen really closely, alleviating some of my fear of being in a car. I am hoping for alleviation from feelings of violation, shame and my ominous fear of the highway as well.

From my journal 5–23–09 (I had some of my journal edited for a short period in a panic when I realized how bad my writing was, and this note is edited):

I do still cower down and hug into myself with my eyes closed tight as I freeze if I am beside any truck the size of a van or larger. I hang on with a death grip to the door and seat for dear life. I have a few guidelines individuals are carrying out for me while driving with me in the car. I have to be in the first or fourth lanes so that traffic is only on one side. I cannot pass a truck or quickly have my driver pass a vehicle on the highway, and a few more idiosyncrasies. Jay leaves about seven car lengths between him and the car next and puts his emergency flashes on when he sees the brake lights of the car ahead, to warn the car behind that we are slowing down. I use back roads at all costs. I have a sense of hopelessness and emptiness for the future and have apparently detached from most people. My passion is gone.

Journal entry 5–27–09 (also edited):

I have a very sensitized startle response, for which I nearly jump out of my skin when hearing a loud noise. The sound of the crash resonates to the echo of a shotgun, a chilling sound from my past. The boom became a major trigger for me as a truck backfiring, screeching of brakes, a door closing, then became my air conditioner turning on, the furnace, the dogs barking, even someone just coming up behind me or hands clapping. Angry outbursts and irritability abound. I am hyper-vigilant. Interference occurs in my relationships, day-to-day functioning and other activities.

My past flashbacks and dreams have re-emerged and intertwined with the most recent events. Recurring nightmares from the past are haunting me in the present.

Dreams

A description from my journal:

> *Frantic, I wake up in a sweat petrified with. Heart pounding, palpitating. Fear trying to find glasses. I have to find. I have switch to using my good arm. Pain shooting down right arm. When move it to feel for my glasses. The rotator cuff pain. I am falling downward, downward, and then my hand touches the case. my glasses are actually in case beside me on night table. Whew, I realize must be having one the car accident dreams.*

I elevate the temporary hospital bed because I cannot transfer into my regular bed with my shoulder out of commission. I have only one good limb to use. I fumble to put my glasses on. I struggle to catch my breath and exercise deep breathing to slow down my heart rate. I am dripping with sweat.

I have these dreams sometimes several times per night. I am in a nondescript car. I get a flash of the highway and then a flash of an accident scene, which I don't see clearly or recognize as my second car crash. I feel very nauseous and cold. I hear the loud crash. My head feels like it is being crushed in a vice. Anxiety consumes me as I feel a jolt. I continue on the highway and then turn into a violent spin – I am hit. I re-experience my first car crash now to the letter. Spinning, spinning, spinning. I hear my thoughts verbatim of knowing I am going to die and flashes of my life. I am spinning and flying across the highway. I am hit again and career across the other way. I see light flashes as I am thrown around in my car between my seat, steering wheel, console and driver's door. Did I just go downward off the highway? It looks like fire. I am sweating profusely, burning up. I feel engulfed in flames. I instantly wake up in the same part of the nightmare. My heart is racing, and my head is pounding. I am soaking wet. I *am* nauseous as I whipped around in my car.

In the first car crash, I landed in the third lane, facing ongoing traffic when the spinning stopped. A sign of the times, I was not wearing a seatbelt. I was thrown around so much between my door and slightly reclined seat back, console and steering wheel. As I flopped all around inside, I saw bits and pieces of light, darkness and fiery colors. I was haunted by those blazing bits of colors and did not know where I was. There was a ledge. I was moving all around and so fast, and the impacts were so loud. I did not know if I had gone over the edge. It took several years before I came to know those fiery colors were bits of sun I was seeing from many angles, and the speed of the car gave them motion, making it look like a roaring blaze in those nightmares. A sign appearing also to be in flames read something like Rte. 128 one mile, which is where I was headed in both instances. My past has forced its way into my present and merged with my only sketchy memories of the second crash.

Other Dreams

While trying to function daily, I have a few other nightmares that prey on my mind – words from nightmares that came out in poetic verse after the first car crash. Back then, while trying to manage the frightful, out-of-my-control nightmares and flashbacks, I tried to tire my mind before going to bed. I worked my way through jigsaw puzzles – some double-sided and another with all the same shape of a complex picture, but to no avail. Nightmares were plentiful as sleep was not. I activated my mind with crossword puzzles, crypto-grams, anagrams, word problems and long-division math problems with letters that I had to convert into numbers.

Still not sleeping, I felt compelled to write down some of my thoughts, usually around two o'clock in the morning, which turned out to be feelings. It started with a few words which I hastily deleted from my computer due to the intense nature. On a notepad, my thoughts and fears elaborated, which I threw away, symbolic of expelling the foreboding feelings. Expressively, text spilled out in poetic verse of darkness and death and started to alleviate my ago-nizing mind. These poems/nightmares have returned.

Dreams

I don't like to dream
I'll tell you why.
The scenes that I see
Make me want to cry.

My demons are here
How they laugh and they crow,
"over the edge you'll go
To an endless nightmare below."

Crashing through the rail
And over the edge
In a dive bomb position
No longer on ledge.

Falling and spinning
And whirling around,
Trapped in a vehicle
That cannot be found.

Flickers and flames
And flashes of light,
I close my eyes
But they're still in sight.

The sign growing larger
And meaner and in flames
Is flashing and rushing
To catch me again.

I strain to scream out
Not a sound could you hear,
But those demons laughing loudly
"How much more can you bear?"

(Genetti, 1992)

Nighttime Fright

I am petrified.
I am scared to death.
I lay here in bed
Clenching hands, holding my breath.

The loud noise outside
I can hear it rush.
It terrifies me
Turns my brain into mush.

The cars racing by
The trucks are there, too.
 I hear the backfire –
The shot 'most blew me in two.'

The cars sound so fast
My head spins the same,
 Then the flashing starts
I see the car and me in flame.

The shivers up my spine
The knowing I am dead.
 I can't get control of
This dizzy pattern in my head.

When will this horror end?
I can't take one more night.
 The accident flashbacks
Will be the death of me by fright.

(Genetti, 1992)

Vividly frightening, nightly nightmares greatly impact my sleeping pattern, causing me to wake at least hourly when I do fall asleep. Consequently, my mood is affected. I am at times irritable and at times so fatigued I can barely comprehend, never mind trying to respond. I captured my inability to speak about my horror in a poem penned in a writing class in 2015:

A Supreme Insidious Ache

No one felt the angst and wretchedness inside her,
eyes closed tight; fists clenched resolutely
A cry drifts in the air
Reverberating from within
Tears spill from her eyes, rolling down
her cheeks and the salty taste
rolls past her now moistened lips.

Arising from the dense fog, she
senses the heaviness of the
darkness cloaking around her body.
She screams a visceral sound as it

emits from her navel
through her abdomen up to her chest
where her breasts lurch forward, fills her
esophagus and then roaring
past her throat, over her tongue and out of
her open mouth, raging like a locomotive.
The tiny silent voice
Resounded – still, no words.
   (Dee Genetti 6–25–15 Writing Grief)

And one more nightmare poem:

Fear

Oh, how I fear cars,
the roadways and byways,
the trucks and the vans.
and interstate highways.

Fear grips my stomach,
flips me into a panic.
I can't live a life
while feeling so manic.

Inside I can't hide
even trapped as I am,
'cause the sounds all around –
I am constantly damned.

Route 93 noise –
and inside motors too –
make me crazy inside
slowly cracking me in two.

The sound of a shot
rings loudly in my head,
the accident sound –
makes me want to be dead.

The flashing of light,
signs larger on the ground,
these visions I see
are distorted – upside down.

Everywhere I look
things are out of place,
crooked and distorted –
I can no longer look and face.

In the outside world,
a rider on the road,
nothing looks the same;
I'm so nauseous and cold.

Everything comes at me –
from cars, trucks and vans,
to people walking in malls,
to trees slanted on the land.

Faster and faster
These images do pass.
With all this distortion
How much longer can I last?

I fear I am crazy.
I know I will crack;
Impulses to stop this
Will cause me to react.

The reaction I've fought,
so hard and so brave,
is winning the battle –
it will end in my grave.

(Genetti, 1992)

With all of these speed bumps hurled in my way, my progress has been halted.

14 Ruts in the Road

Reckoning with Anger

Around October 2009, through my therapist, I become aware that my daily life is vacillating. It is between languishing with severe depression and irateness with sudden angry outbursts leaping out, many times without merit. This is symptomatic of both TBI and PTSD. Fluctuating between what Ellie deemed as rage and despair, totally against my composition, I cannot express my emotions appropriately.

From my journal 10–6–09:

> I haven't been able to write here for a while. I hit my desk very hard with fist. Four small rubber balls and a rubber smiley face to throw – I was in receipt of from my occupational therapist. I threw very hard at wall – felt good to get energy out physically, but scary. Also paced in my chair up and down hall a lot but didn't get enough energy out.

From journal entry 10–09–09:

> Hurt hand with bang on desk. Throw balls didn't do it. I screamed viscerally – really helped get some of the negative energy out. Very emotional, very sad, very depressed, strong suicidal ideation. I screamed from my navel several times as loud as I could with no one else around. It started at my navel, moved up to my abdomen into my chest – I did it again -felt better- the tiny silent voice inside erupted.

Other episodes include: loud and raging screams with the stereo on, progressing into a more civilized loud singing. *Cry Baby* by Janis Joplin is sung particularly loud, especially with Ellie while on the phone. Additionally, I slam my fist into a wooden gate, and then

DOI: 10.4324/9781003428510-18

again, for civility, I obtain a rubber mallet. The negative energy has
to come out some way and safely.

Journal entry 10–16–09:

> *Sudden – feels like pent up energy – but hasn't been building – suddenly*
> *very, very angry/frenzy feeling – just going to explode – more, can't*
> *describe – and tell it like it f – g really is – in the moment.*

And from my journal entry 10–22–09:

> *All revved up, can't stand these feelings – was total despair then*
> *antsy?? – can't describe – want to put myself out of my misery, all feel-*
> *ings – jumbled – can't leave windows open – love fresh air – highway*
> *below/behind too noisy, triggering – can't stand it – flips me – flashing*
> *. . .*
>
>   *Angry outburst – can't figure to dry my hair – revved up then*
> *crying – crying more tears than in my whole life . . .*
>   *Can't stand myself – being with me – feeling – can't sit in my skin*
> *. . . speedy, speedy, speedy – gonna explode, went to kitchen and read*
> *post-it notes on cabinets – reminders, bring me back to the present –*
> *All around kitchen post-it notes to remind me to stop and not react.*
> *"that was then, this is now;" "you're safe, it's over now;" "no impulses"*
> *with a circle around and a line going through it; "call a particular*
> *friend" who said she would be available at any time and was; and*
> *other reminders "don't off the b – " posted on cabinets, including my*
> *"going out the door list.* End journal entry.

In late October 2009, I am clinging to hope that Dr. Jacob and Dr.
Chi will have a magical answer as they review my whole spectrum
of assessments. I think they will say, "This is where/what you are,
this is where you can get to, and this is how you can get there." I
am still ready and willing to put in the work, but everything else
seems to be spilling out of me. They conclude I need a doctor
who specializes in both TBI and PTSD. Both diagnoses are new in
the field and just coming into awareness as co-occurring disorders.
Searching for someone credentialed in both is exceptionally difficult. It takes a few more months. Finally finding such a person in
great demand, I go back into rehab. I am clinging to life by holding
onto my short-length, anything-but-hard fingernails, slowly scraping down the wall. By now, I have no tolerance, still have angry
outbursts, and I still cannot articulate, which is now coming out in
g-d-f-g expletives.

From my journal entry 11–12–09:

> *too tired to think of dinner . . . Othello wants go for walk – I remember now why I don't take him for walks with just me – the block – I ran out of f – in g – d – power – my wheelchair battery died part way around the circle – I forgot to friggin charge my chair last night too. neighbor switched me to manual overdrive – pushed me back home- thankful for. I hate having to have someone with me all the having a really bad day today. can't even sort laundry – can't decide what colors go – I've been doing for about a hundred years – sat for about an hour trying to do – what the hell????? I have no quALITY of my life – depressing. Rolled away defeated. What the heck??? I have no quality of my life – depressing. I don't have my life, my life has me.*
> > *– some days I just almost don't even know my name*

Of note, on 12–1–09, I had my second shoulder surgery. It will be six to eight weeks in a sling to heal. A later journal entry:

> *I cried today – new thoughts – I'm still back in June in time – it's really 14 days before Christmas – this has always been my favorite – haven't even thought of it at all*

Journal entry 1–4–10:

> *No tolerance – can't modulate – flipping out between g d f-ing rage and f-ing despair – NOTHING IN BETWEEN*
> *– CAN'T TAKE THE F-ING FLASHBACKS*
> *– SUICIDAL F-ING FEELINGS – WHAT THE F IS THAT ABOUT – CAN'T F-ING*
> *GET RID OF THEM*
> *– CAN'T THEM – RAGE HELPS ME NOT TO ACT ON THEM F-ING SUICIDAL FEELINGS FROM F-ING BEFORE, WHAT THE F – AND NOW SO MUCH RAGE INSIDE – WHAT THE F DO I DO WITH THESE FEELINGS – CAN'T STAND IT – CAN'T STAND MY F-ING SELF*
> *– HARD SITTING WITH EITHER END OF THESE FEELINGS – RAGE OR DESPAIR*
> *AT LEAST RAGE GIVES ME ENERGY BETTER TO FIGHT OTHER FEELINGS OFF – BUT TOO F-ING LONG – I CAN'T GO ON LIKE THIS – BIGGGGGGGGGGGG FUCKING SCREAMMMMMMMMMMM.*

Despair, despondent – not a speck of energy – don't want to be here – prolonging terrible agony, anguish, misery, non-stop

Another entry:

THE F-ING DEPRESSION IS SO DEEP – I DON'T KNOW HOW TO HELP MYSELF – IS BEYOND MY CAPACITY NOW – CAN'T LIVE IN MY SKIN – CAN'T THINK ANY NORMAL THOUGHTS
– WHAT THE F IS EVEN A NORMAL THOUGHT – BEEN SUNK UNDER HERE FOR SO LONG NOW
– FEEL HUGE F-ING WEIGHT – FEEL BURRIED ALIVE – HEAVY WEIGHT ON TOP OF ME – VERY VERY F-ING DARK PLACE – NO F-ING LIGHT – HARD TO F-ING BREATHE
– this is me – I am suffering.

How much can one person really take, I wonder. I am so tired and feel so old – how many times can I learn everything all over?????? I have searched and perceived new gains emotionally, spiritually, and even physically through my many trials in life . . . I used to feel the saying, "Life is a verb." Now, it isn't even a noun to me. Every nerve ending feels exposed and pains – even my oversized light shirt seems to hurt wherever barely scraping my skin.

Journal entry 1–6–10:

I'M SO FREAKING TIRED AND TIRED OF BEING TIRED. I am ready for forever sleep.
    Put CD in computer – mammas & pappas – one I like relaxing – Filled with anxiety – too overloaded – big time – Lowered volume – all way to barely hearing – listened a bit for few minutes – Then had to turn off altogether – over stimulating – makes anxiety

Exceptionally uncharacteristic of me is this journal entry: 1–15–10:

Used to be caretaker for everyone – had capacity to hold the whole world – now I can't even hold my own stuff. Some close to me think I'm now just all about me – not available to them. few people who know suicidal ideation that I can't crawl out from feels it's a personal affront on them – what the fuck is wrong with these g d people – get a fucking life with real problems – I no tolerance – just fucking out of control with everybody – talk a bit – short conversations – ok, then

> *too long or too many people calling – no control – people pissing me off – no tolerance for any crap – feel explosive – heart pounding out of chest.*

Astonishingly unlike me are these thoughts, emotional reactions and language! I should be horrified; instead, I feel diminished, debilitated, demoralized. What would seem like forever sleep, which I desperately need, is a difficult dream about death that I struggle deeply to free myself from.

As I observe my enduring suffering at this juncture, I neither witness nor feel any positive growth from my traumatic brain injury. As others have claimed, I have not been blessed in any way with this brain injury. I have to re-evaluate my every belief, assumption, purpose, value, function and direction of my life. My new limitations have no new positive meaning that I can find. Just prior to the car crash, I was working on my life's purposes (I had two), which I had already discovered. I felt it fully in my heart and soul, and it was fulfilling. I had a balance or a tendency to be overworked . . . but I was happy, content without being complacent, and accomplished, radiating inside and out. My cup, at that time, was more than half full. My cup runneth over. My cup is now empty.

15 Breakdown Lane

Impatient rehabilitation

My personal vulnerability is exposed. I do not feel capable or even worthy of anything anymore. Do I want to continue living in this unpredictable and dangerous world where life can be taken away from me at any time? Where life is confusion daily? I am being pushed beyond my limits, over the barrier, headlong . . . now decelerating . . . debilitating . . . disintegrating on death's door. Suicidal ideation ingrained deeply consumes me. From whence did it come – a symptom of TBI? PTSD? MDD? Medication side effect? All viable disorders – it could be a combination of all of the above. It is diagnosed as "mood disorder after TBI." I have hung on for as long as I can possibly persist.

Consumed in total despair lay I here. I feel the unbearable, unstoppable, tensing ache that churns in the pit of my stomach when I have the strength to even comprehend a thought about my ruin. I have been battling these dreadful feelings for quite some time. Having been depressed before, I feel this much deeper still, into the bowels of the earth, dark, dank and cold, completely isolated. I hear the black wrath of death drawing me near. My parched lips experience the bad taste in my acrid mouth. Darkness abounds. My light is but a fading flicker.

In-patient Therapies

It takes four months for me to get an appointment with my new doctor specializing in both TBI and PTSD. Under dire straits, I am admitted in-patient into a rehabilitation hospital under his care, which isn't until April 2010. My care includes physical, language and cognitive therapies, occupational therapy training in coping skills and to manage rage and pharmacology for PTSD and depression/suicidality from 4–20–10 to 5–19–10. The physical therapist

DOI: 10.4324/9781003428510-19

works on my right shoulder, neck, head and arm on one day and range of motion exercises with my legs the next day for continued stretching to prevent loss in the range of motion, stiffness and rigidity. While speech and language therapy conduct their own individual assessments, pharmacology tries out medications and doses daily, and then there is occupational therapy, which is very different.

My self-observations reveal the use of occupational group sessions, including my participation in visual guided imageries. I capture some in my journal and work on them on my own. In my room, I conjure up images of a beach with calming blue waters or the forest with the inviting waft of the pine cones, sap and trees with the light brown blanket of needles below my wheels and the quietness imposed all around with the exception of birds chirping, and other quiet and calming places I find within myself. Performing relaxation exercises is taking place. Deep breathing ensues. Lavender sprinkled on Q-tips lay in with the chips on sachet packets wrapped in lace with tiny purple bows that I brought from home, the scent almost gone. Lifting the sachet closer, I deep breathe in the fragrance of serenity as I gently rub the satin beneath the lace between my thumb and my forefinger. It is very calming and peaceful. I can hear the soothingness of the total quiet; nothing going on in my head – just complete relaxation. **Then a door bangs, and I am in a flashback again. I jump, quite shaken by hearing the startling sound.**

I participate in individual occupational therapy sessions in my room. I am assisted with tactile balls to finger in my hands when I feel anger starting to arise. If that does not ease, I am instructed to throw them firmly against the wall as hard as I can, along with several rubber balls to squeeze and throw. One has a smiley face, which I find antagonistic when I feel an angry outburst. Scrunching it in my fist, I hurl it at the wall, where it just bounces to the side. Seems pointless. Punching or crying into a pillow is allowable. I also have custom, accommodating activities, most of which are beyond my memory at this time.

In the occupational therapy room in this hospital, filled with colorful bins of various exercise gear, computers and other assistive equipment, as well as books and handouts, I sit in my wheelchair at a hefty table. Dressed in a long, jean skirt with a nondescript oversized tee shirt, my hands neatly folded in my lap, I wait. The room of all off-white walls has a floor with no carpet, which is easier for my wheelchair to roll on. Seated beside me is Topher, my occupational therapist.

It is April 30, 2010. I hear Topher, the OT, speaking in a louder and purposeful tone. He shockingly tells me straight out and boldly, in words I have not heard, "You are judging yourself too harshly from where you used to be. You were a different person, one that you will never be again." He goes on, "It is time to give up the 'old you.'" Topher tells me he will not allow me to speak about the "old me," and names specifically my work, schooling and counseling, committees and anything that used to define who I *was*. He tells me to develop new interests and meet people who know my brain now and have nothing to compare it to. Even my new doctor says, "We have to find you a new purpose." It sounds cavalier to me, like it should be easy to do just that, without any emotional baggage, or so it seems to me at this point in time. This is so close to me. It cuts deep into my heart, feeling like it leaves me oozing with blood and tears.

My biggest fear at the moment is that I will now lose all of me. So much has vanished. I do not want to grieve and find new interests. I like my old interests passionately, even though I cannot keep up the pace with necessary activities, and my associates, who are caring, but have a job to do, hence have gone forward without me. I am several steps behind, actually neighborhoods behind by now. Topher tells me to "develop new hobbies and interests." He continues that position for the duration of my hospital stay, trying to outwardly push me into making a weekly plan for when to try new things. I feel deflated, depleted, denied and confused about who I am and who I am evolving into. This generates more anger but then causes me to go deeper into myself.

During this time in the hospital, my lifetime of traumas caught up with me. I remember resilience triumphing for me from untold horror episodes in my childhood to then being out on my own in my tender teens. I married when I turned 20 and started running a successful business. I had a three-year-old and a one-year-old and was running my businesses when I was hit by a van taking an illegal turn on the highway. I am, again, seeing the huge tire as it turns and comes straight at my driver's window, slamming right into me – a haunting scene. I *feel* the depression I experienced back then and severe flashbacks and symptoms of PTSD following the accident.

I vividly recall the first accident, both pre- and post-car crash. I am seeing and feeling it frequently. I am traveling in the first lane of I-93 South, about 55 miles per hour, at about one mile before my exit. I am in my five-week-old two-toned platinum and fox silver with black pinstriping Datsun 280ZX 2+2. With the T-roofs removed, the windows up, and a warm breeze from the 75-degree day, the wind brushes softly against my cheek as it tosses my bangs up and to the side. The scent of newness of the soft, contoured leather seats fill my nostrils as the Eagles sing out in concert from the five-speaker Dolby surround sound system custom-installed. I know I am on my way to my office after dropping off my son, who has just been cleared at his very first well-baby check-up at the age of 12 months. He has been very sickly this first year of life with critical ailments. I can feel life at this time is good. I am innocent, minding my business and following the rules of the road. I barely have time to register that I see the big tire taking a right-hand turn, coming straight for my driver's side window with no time to react. Bang!!!! The flash-back continues with the dizzying pattern and confusing fiery light shapes I have previously described. The driver is given traffic cita-tions for reckless driving, illegally crossing the line on the highway, not using his blinker and speeding – and walks away. I remember that part clearly. I don't have a clear visual of the second car crash. I do have the bodily sensations.

Integrating Memory

Out in the larger social context, I find the prevailing cognitive mod-els of treatment for symptoms of PTSD recovery. That is for an indi-vidual to contextualize their experience and feel safe, integrating the traumatic memory into one's autobiographical memory base and allowing for a coherent narrative of their experience. I also find that integrating trauma memories into memory is difficult due to the way in which they are encoded. Under conditions of extreme arousal, the encoding of experiences is fragmented, causing a disturbance in the capability to shape the essential coherent narrative. In the context of TBI, fragmented memories of the traumatic occurrence can happen due to impaired consciousness secondary to the injury. One of the complexities of treating PTSD after TBI is the patient's capability to reconstruct traumatic events in a coherent, adaptive way. Or even to accept the vagueness of how events happened when they suffered their TBI. This may interfere with their ability to draw a context of the occurrence into their autobiographical memory base.

My Path Moving Forward

I come out of rehab on 5–19–10 . . . still confused, but stronger holistically. Rick's progress note for my visit on 5–26–10, one week later, triangulates where I am at in this timeframe:

Patient remains tangentially mildly verbose with significantly downed working memory. Patient loses train of thought several times. Needs cues to verbalize, as memory placeholder. Overall, markedly less agitation and also improved attention and memory, yet the cognitive area remains crippling.

I have a lot to work on, which includes cognition, depression and even though suicidal feelings are more in control, it takes time before they alleviate. In the future (November, 2015) in a writing class, I penned words to the relief I feel when I finally am able to let go, which I couldn't verbalize in this timeframe:

I Did Not Go

I did not say good-bye.
    I didn't really want to go. But the
        sea sucked me into a rip current. Whirling
        in its grip I struggled to keep my head
    above water. Gurgling
and gasping.
Gurgling
    and gasping.
        I churned around and around and around.
        Then I stopped
    the fight and just let go.
I just let go.
    The sea dragged me to the rocky shore.
        I did not go.
I did not need to say good-bye.

Spiritual Decline

For the next year, into my fourth year post-TBI, I have a very difficult time. Brooding and pondering manifest. The very core of my spiritual life is flipped upside down, sideways and inside out when I am able to think long enough. In my human frailty, I question my faith, especially regarding fate. I renounced my faith back and forth for quite some time. Pondering Topher's comments about a new identity, I seek out the strengthening of hope. I seek out the creation of a sense of meaning and purpose and access to my intuition. I am trying to have faith, but the primal understanding of my dilemma is nowhere within my reach or understanding. And what is fate anyway?

It is 2011, the fourth year post-TBI. As I sit in front of my healing altar, I feel the cool touch of the green Connemara marble
pocket rosary beads given to me during my pilgrimage in Knock,
Ireland (and as well to Lourdes, France), draped around one hand.
I light the candles with a lighter in the other. I have been coming
here quite frequently. With low light, they illuminate my special
place. I can smell the bayberry candle burning and underneath
the smell of the cedar wood I used to make the altar, with its
natural knots and holes where light from the window above peaks
through. From my journal, my ruminative brooding and pondering on 4–12–11:

> *I wonder how this could possibly happen – so deeply – again. my
> biggest fear now – I don't want to face a questioning meaning
> to another tragic event -not again – anger surges. how could God
> want this to happen to me? How could He possibly choose another
> route to disability – again? Of course I want to find meaning. I try
> to believe this just a bad thing that happened – I was in the wrong
> place at the wrong time – not fate but happenstance – when bad
> things happen to good people – maybe thinking – things happen and
> God gives us hope and the strength to make it through – if we access
> our faith and search . . . I could not believe that my God would be
> so cruel as to have another severe, permanent injury and for what
> purpose could there be to justify or merit this end – I wish I had
> my [articulate] mind to think through . . . I have searched and
> perceived new growth emotionally and spiritually, even physically
> through my many trials in life. Why would God put me through
> all of this? How much can just one person take? This IS more than
> I handle. Why me – again? I want to be able to think.*

On 5–1–11, my journal entry reveals my thoughts:

> *I found new meaning – changed course of my life in first acci-
> dent – always knew I had a purpose since a child – found my life's
> purpose several times – which felt right- though not my ultimate
> purpose. I did find my ultimate purpose when began working with
> trauma especially with those with PTSD [from physical and sexual
> abuse, in childhood and adulthood] and those with co-occurring
> substance abuse. I knew – I felt it – that was my calling.*

I hung onto that feeling in a tight grasp on my narrow mental
clipboard.

My journal entry of 6–10–11:

> *I worked hard to recover and could find no good – felt helpless and hopeless, my faith waning, my passion gone, my inner light faint. another huge obstacle to overcome in order to become the whole me, to travel another path on my journey through life – the path less taken or is it the road to nowhere? who am I now resulting from my TBI? who am I meant to be? . . . with grace and dignity – – well grace and dignity ain't happening.*

Rumination persists. I do not have enough cognitive functioning and available brain space to work this out at this time. On 6–23–11:

> *I feel I have gone backwards and lost so much I cannot even say. I struggled with the value of my life for so long. I haven't had appreciation each day – many days are just a blur. Are my days justifiable if all I have done is make it through the day alive? After first accident I saw how life could be cut so short. I tried to live my life to the fullest. That is not possible now – I have much fewer possibilities at this level.*

Shattered Assumptions

I do not fully subscribe to or accept that this is the way it is now. I do not feel that my life is better or that I am a better person for having a brain injury, as some with post-traumatic growth have said. I haven't found, as many with PTG report, that any good has come out of this accident nor any new opportunities, new interests or better prospects at the expense of a new disability. My outlook has become cynical. From my journal 7–20–11:

> *I have already done this before and do not have a feeling of glowing happiness to do it yet again. It's getting tougher.*

In November of 2011, I become more aware of the breadth of my shattered self. I have not been able to maintain a sense of identity – any identity. My sense of good has been crushed. How could this have happened? Can I ever be repaired? Now that this has happened, how can I do any good in the world? How can I be restored to wholeness? How can certain or any fairness happen in the world – my world? Are we, am I, destined to be victims of external events, to lose our sense of freedom over our destiny to wallow in anger, fear and anxiety? My sense of self collapses in view of the emotions of anguish, anger and fear. With a rigid identity, I identify strongly with one of my identities, which is in the society of those with TBI and PTSD. Anger arises as emotions settle from sitting with the fear of the unknown, grief and ambiguity. Anger is suppressed when anxiety, fear and anguish are in the forefront of the mind. These emotions loop over and over as I contemplate my existence. My mind is now starting to expand with more capacity to hold and understand. My writing and continued work with Rick in cognitive therapy, which is difficult, is working out and stretching my brain. I am struggling with the issues of how to incorporate and negotiate new identities associated with TBI: survivor of this traumatic experience, woman with a disability, disabled woman with another disability, mother with a new disability and adjustment to brain injury. Am I to leave the breakdown lane? Am I ready to merge into another lane or will I be ducking in and out of lanes unknown?

Trek Three

Petals Opening One by One: Changing Lanes

Years 5 and 6 Post-TBI: Changes in Philosophy of Life: Acceptance of My New Life

16 At the Cross Roads
Spiritual Crisis

In this fifth and sixth year (2012, 2013), I find my *new normal*. I progress on the Rancho Los Amigos Recovery scale to Level VIII marked as:

> **purposeful, appropriate**, needing standby assistance. The patient is independent for familiar tasks in a distracting environment for one hour. He or she acknowledges impairments but has difficulty self-monitoring. Emotional issues such as depression, irritability and low frustration tolerance may be observed. Abstract reasoning abilities are decreased relative to pre-morbid levels.
>
> (Hagen et al., 1972, para 8)

I am amid a terrible spiritual and moral crisis. I have come through my process of figuring out what to do through the phases of adjustments, including my foggy unawareness and loss of self-perception. I have come through the process of figuring out how to live by meeting Rick and by becoming aware of the ramifications of TBI and PTSD. As well I have come through by feeling my losses and suicidal ideation and learning how to re-establish relationships. Now, in this timeframe, I am trying to figure out the meaning of my struggle. I seem to go through Kubler-Ross's (1997) Acceptance stage of grief, which is characterized as an individual beginning to come to terms with her mortality or inevitable future. This stage comes with a calm, retrospective view and a stable mindset. I do not go through the third stage of Bargaining, nor do I go through grief in linear stages. I definitely grieve my traumatic losses, though, especially my loss of self. Some criticize Kubler-Ross (1997), arguing that most people who experience a loss do not grieve, but are resilient. They claim

DOI: 10.4324/9781003428510-21

that the main component of grief and trauma reactions is natural resilience. It is my belief, however, as a psychologist and a mourner, that resilience is the outcome of grief after loss.

From my reflective and process journals, I see that I go through a process to search for the meaning and personal significance of my traumatic event. With a longer independent focus ability of about one hour, I can focus on my perceptions and beliefs. It is difficult, though, since my abstract reasoning is still quite decreased. My perceptions and beliefs have changed to my very core. I am, however, able to realize that certain likelihoods in my life will never become possibilities. I begin to look for ways in which to reconfigure my goals. This involves constructs of cognitive appraisals (thinking), which include ruminative brooding, reflective pondering with intrusive and avoidant thoughts and a few other cognitive activities. As well I question the level of centrality, which is the extent to which an individual believes a negative event has become a part of their essence.

Through my research, I am reminded that a high level of post-traumatic stress leading to a probable diagnosis of PTSD is likely to mean that an individual's coping ability is challenged. This is where I have been. My ability to process cognitively and work through my trauma is impeded. However, I am starting to use more constructive cognitive processing. This is evident when I ruminate about the car crash, its significance and what sense can become of it. This thinking is associated with post-traumatic growth.

Low levels of growth and high levels of distress have been my path, indicative of ruminations. These thoughts have been primarily negative, intrusive and have persisted unabated for wide-ranging periods of time. Like others in the broader society, I feel that my relationships, my visions of the world and my good judgment of myself have been crushed. My thought process is cycling from ruminative brooding, reflective pondering and coping. Through revising and rebuilding my assumptions, the possibility of growth is more comprehensible. An epiphany strikes: individuals who try to put their lives back the way they were remain vulnerable and fractured. However, individuals who accept the breakage and rebuild themselves become more resilient and open to new ways of living. I am smack in the middle of these two frames.

Many trauma survivors experience positive psychological experiences after trauma, even though the experience of trauma can, for years, go together with severe psychological distress and emotional experience. I have found this personally and now professionally.

Ambivalence and Rumination

Traumatic events trigger ruminative brooding or thinking. Intrusive rumination is unwanted thoughts of the traumatic event recurring while not trying to think about it. Deliberate rumination is thinking about the event purposefully and relating it to growth. This happens through anticipation, problem-solving, making sense and reminiscing. The result is PTG (post-traumatic growth), which appears as finding meaning. I am stuck in ruminative brooding at this time. I am failing to produce any meaning or resolve any discrepancies. However, I do have some processing happening. It causes me to think about my past experiences and assumptions with the new trauma information. This includes my first car crash and injuries, my personhood, the way I saw the world and this new car crash and injuries with my pessimistic view of the world.

From my journal 2–7–12, I find myself thinking:

> *what if . . . I left ten minutes later, . . . I decided not to go to the mall that day, . . . we went the back roads which I did frequently.*

This pattern plays as a loop in my head that reinforces negative emotional states such as anger, guilt, shame and rage. Reflective pondering makes its way in here, which brings about the positive emotion of hope and a bit of optimism, but joy and other positive emotions reflective of post-traumatic growth do not factor in at this time.

Caught also in my ruminating loop from my journal on 2–12–12:

> *I did not deserve to be hit again or to have another devastating accident. I had lost enough in my diminutive view. I do not accept the reasons others give me for why this happened to me. Did I discover that I am stronger than I thought I was? I almost lost my life. I borrowed the strength from several people close to me, including my therapist Ellie and Dr. Bob. I just hung on by a thread and had lost my faith in my abilities and God.*

In the adjustment to TBI and PTSD, I am finding the following three questions to be common: Why did this happen to me? Will I be normal again? Is life worth living after brain injury? The latter two are brooding within me. This is continuing my, albeit slow, quest for meaning. I found that distress may motivate some individuals to search for meaning and direction in their lives.

I am very angry with God, with random acts and with men at this time, as both crashes were the fault of men. I am mad at the world, and I guess at myself for not being able to get back to me. I have a new me, but I really liked the old me, the real me, and my life with great satisfaction. I am so isolated now and have such a drudgery getting through my days. I work tremendously for my recovery, but I do not know that I am going to recover any further than I have. My brain injury undermines my sense of hope and spiritual belief that if I work hard and live a "good life," then I will be at peace.

My thinking shifts from brooding to pondering. My ability to communicate, though, is opening. This is especially happening through my continued cognitive work with Rick and broadening my focus ability. I am more able to ponder reflectively. This helps me to move even more toward aiding in the resolution between my prior assumptions and new negative trauma-related informational worlds.

Assimilation and accommodation processes are happening. Some of my discrepancies are starting to resolve. I am realizing that by retaining my pre-existing assumptions and yearning to be back to my old self, there is potential for further traumatization. This would happen following any new trauma exposure, should my world remain unchanged. With my damaged memory, I have also forgotten much of what I was trying to get back to. I am reminded when I reread my resume, which I still have on my desktop. Also, the burning desire for achievement that I have had most of my life since I was a child has fizzled. This is both a blessing and a curse.

In March 2012 and throughout this fifth year post-TBI, I find that I am able to go deeper into myself, search and ultimately come out again with another vision. I have to fearlessly face my fateful dilemma. When I feel I can go on no longer, I put my fate back into the hands of God. I am lifted up. I find a bit of serenity, which gives me a quiet sense of power. It liberates my spirit. I am reminded that I view my body as a container for my sacred spirit so that it is protected and able to act in the world. I recognize, though, that I need to reinforce self-care. Realizing that we are more than our bodies, I feel my spirit helps in coping with ultimate mortality. I view my body as a pathway to provide a way to access my spiritual resources.

Listening to my journal on 6–9–12, I recognize that in critical moments, I have always accessed my spirit. I am eventually able to make my way through a small clearing in my foggy maze to realize that my spiritual dimension strengthens my trust in myself and others. This happens through my relationship with God, through my participation in the community of the spirit and in my interactions with Robert, my Eucharistic Minister and spiritual advisor. Robert has been coming weekly for more than fourteen years. We say the prayers of a Mass, and he gives me communion. Robert also brings blessings to my house and current parish information. We have in-depth spiritual conversations and talks of our families. I reincorporate my spiritual resources into my daily life, including commitment to the right actions (suicide not being one of them). They include: spiritual enlightenment with Robert and, at times, with our pastor, and performing my personal rituals, one of which is the spiritual power of the Rosary. Lifting my heart a bit definitively helps with my depression and feelings of being lost.

In my pondering, I realize that before the second car crash, I had attained an indescribable and nonverbal sense of high connectedness with God. This involved acceptance, compassion and love for myself and others. My old mantra reveals that through God, I have moments of clarity. They help me to understand the nature of life, the meaning of my past, and the purpose of my future. There is a lot more to life than the material world. I have always been keenly aware of this, especially arising from my recovery from several major life adversities. Remembering this mantra, which does not resonate with me at the moment, I continue actions of ruminative brooding and reflective pondering.

On 6–29–12 from my journal:

> *meditative message from the [church] bulletin today: you are blessed with the gift of life which was bestowed on you by God.*

This message comes to me at just the right time. I realize my life is not of my own but is truly a gift to cherish and care for from God. I lift my arms and put myself in the hands of God. I regain a semblance of hope. I am still trying to get back to some measure of my old life. Through soul searching, I realize if I remain fixated on these thoughts, the probability of progressing to the next higher level of functioning will be slight. I am forced to alter deeply my ingrained ways of interacting with the world. I must question my fundamental beliefs and worldviews. With this, I may be able to change my forethoughts into a more positive light. I eventually become empowered to slowly shed my negative views. It is difficult as my mind is still slow at multiple functions. I am still one step at a time.

While able to hold a few more thoughts in my head at a time, I become more aware that my life *has* changed significantly. I am now consciously aware that I have to reconsider my viewpoints rather than relying on instinctive or unconscious motivations. This will hopefully allow me to change my behavior to the extent my brain injury can permit. I am finding strength and guidance through my prayers and meditations of the heart, alone and with Robert. I am rethinking my values – what I think is right, good and just. I am rethinking my beliefs about truths that no longer ring true, that I automatically incorporated from childhood and modified after the first accident. I am rethinking morals – my systems of beliefs of right and wrong and habits of conduct that aren't fully inclusive anymore. I find my resilience has been slow in recovering. As I let go of more of what I am holding onto so tightly, my relationship with God strengthens, which feels paradoxical.

In another slight awakening, my mind seems to open more, and I realize my attention and focus is increasing into longer sessions. In July of 2012, I reflectively come to the understanding that it really is a forever road we are on. I note in my journal on 7–18–12:

> *after blindly sitting on the edge of the road in my fog for so many years, I was able to finally roll out a bit and see down the road. Not the end of the road but a new one in the clearing that is yet unpaved. It is a long road/journey, but I am doing it with God right by my side, and at moments, like footprints in the sand, He's carried me when I felt I could not go on.*

My spiritual and religious meaning perspectives have changed. I was confused and distressed. I questioned my faith. I have had Robert to help guide me. He met me at my pace and place, with delicate matters, and does not scorn me. I can talk with him about my doubts as well as some of the depths of my suicidal feelings (mostly spoken about with Ellie). He sits with me in silences. He helps me to reconstruct my meanings that have become discombobulated. Now, a year later, I find that I have a deepening of my spirituality, allowing for areas of answerless mysteries. I also see new possibilities that I did not want to see before, as I wanted my old possibilities back. These are two factors of post-traumatic growth. It helps me with the strengthening of hope, with the creation of a new sense of meaning and purpose (although not fully defined) and access to intuition. I have the feeling of a better understanding of spiritual matters, though not fully resolved. I am developing an even stronger religious faith.

17 Staying the Course
Transcending My Story

In this fifth year post-TBI of 2012, I am progressing to taking a few social actions. This is a step forward for post-traumatic growth. Transcending my story by taking action upon it socially completes the process. The first action occurs as I am accepted back into my PhD program from my leave of absence (!) of almost six years and the writing of my dissertation. I wrote an analytic memo that is being reviewed by my doctoral committee, along with a lot of other considerations. I have remained in close contact with my extraordinary doctoral committee. I feel I am ready, as do they, to start writing my thesis domains and to continue as my focus has evolved. I also welcome a lovely, exceptional new member to my committee, Dr. Julia Byers. She is taking the Chair position as another goes on sabbatical for a short term. Throughout my lengthy time of completing my dissertation, each of these amazing women on my committee, including Dr. Susan Gere and Dr. Caroline Heller, have taken turns on sabbatical, but all are ready at a moment's notice to support me. I am truly blessed.

I continue to write in my exercises with Rick and do other cognitive work for comprehending, verbalizing and attending to material in the context of my professional endeavors. This includes: listening to and taking notes as though at a conference, performing research and understanding research methods and material. As a reasonable accommodation for some of my TBI deficits, I begin working with Dr. Daniel Newman at Lesley University. Dan is another exceptional individual I am blessed with, who tutors me in academic support. We meet individually in April 2012 and then again in May 2012 with my full doctoral committee. Our goal is to talk about what my project will look like and what types of support I will need. This means the world to me. My purpose is back. Dan's background is in understanding graduate and doctoral writing and research papers.

DOI: 10.4324/9781003428510-22

We meet by phone weekly and every now and then in person. We review my dissertation structure and go over organizing and brainstorming concepts together.

I continue to work with Ellie in therapy every two weeks in this timeframe of 2012. We are working on my shattered assumptions, ambivalence, rumination, reflective pondering and rebuilding my new self/my new normal. I go to assistive technology (AT) with Rachael for periods of three months at a time, with breaks in between. I see Rick (ST) every two to three weeks, with a focus on learning and utilizing compensatory cognitive strategies to apply to the writing of my dissertation. I see Dr. Bob every three to four weeks, as he follows my progress closely. Another dear person I am blessed with, Dr. Bob has committed to not letting me fall through the cracks and has been a pillar of strength, encouragement and forward direction for me.

I continue physical therapy for my right arm, pectoral muscles, shoulder and neck, and am receiving cortisone shots in my right shoulder which still has a tear in the rotator cuff. The surgeon has said he knows he can finally resolve my pain through another surgery. I am not willing to face that again, though. At least not right now. I've already been through two surgeries. I see my interpersonal relationships evolving at this point. It is happening especially with Jay, my father and my Aunt Pat. My greatest growth is in trusting them and the people close to me. I am letting them help me even from afar – Atlantic City and Kentucky. I am experiencing post-traumatic growth as I see I am putting more effort into my relationships. I have a willingness to share my emotions and be heard. This is a change from me holding everything in and feeling that no one will be able to understand. My Aunt, especially, is able to hear where I am, even at my lowest. She acknowledges it without judgment. This is validating. And she gives me encouraging words of wisdom that I consider pearls of wisdom and value greatly – each and every day. We have a mutual, incredibly special, close, respectful and deeply loving relationship.

Panel Speaker

With Rick, I have been trying for about the past six months to verbalize an elevator speech of my dissertation. It is a short, concise, complete synopsis that can be stated in the short span of an elevator ride. Condensing any subject into a few words is very difficult for me. I am usually quite verbose. I also do not have it formulated well in my head, in part because it is still developing. In order to help me in this process, Rick invites me to speak on a panel of TBI survivors at Boston University. This is the next step in my rehabilitation. This forces me to connect my present with my past in a cohesive story, which will help my developing self to be more fully realized.

The speaking engagements with honoraria are to Rick's graduate students. They are readying for careers in the field of Speech-Language Pathology. The course is on brain injury rehabilitation. I speak in February 2012 and again in February and June of 2013, in March of 2014 and in April and July of 2015. These speeches take place during fall, spring and summer courses. I make tremendous strides, having to: prepare a speech of sorts, present it in full sentences, ensure it makes sense and remember what it is I want to say. I have to order my experience in the sequence of events – difficult. Relationally, I grow exponentially through these speaking engagements. I relate to the students. A surprising positive consequence happens as I relate with the other panelists. They are all just like me in their need to develop and use compensatory strategies to accomplish everyday tasks due to their brain injuries! And they work! What a relief and sense of camaraderie to meet similar others and not have to explain ourselves to each other. We already know! We understand!

Some of the useful similar strategies others are using are: the use of day planners and other note-taking devices such as notebooks, cell phones, computers, tape recorders, alarm systems and others I cannot remember. I do not write them down at this time for future reference. It is beyond my capacity. I have all I can do to stay focused on my speech. We all have a style of written speech, but all in very different formats and with different deliveries. I have a new assistive tool with me tonight to follow the date and time, as Rick always asks me every time I see him. I finally bought a talking watch. With one press, it tells me the time. With two presses, it tells me the day and date. Now I just have to remember to wear it or put it into my pocketbook.

There are usually three or four other TBI survivor panel members. All of us have attended speech-language and cognitive therapy currently or formerly with Rick. All of us have different levels and various lengths of time since brain injury. The person with the longest time since the injury that I have met is a woman more than ten years into her recovery. We all speak with reference to an agenda from our speeches, cue cards or other notes and note-taking devices that we have prepared for this occasion. Rick prompts us to touch on certain aspects should/when we forget what we are saying. Forgetfulness is a very common symptom of TBI. This proves incalculably helpful in putting us at ease and ensuring that we cover our topics. We all look normal, although we can recognize fatigue in each other when it sets in.

All of us panelists have varying strategies and many of the same problems, even though our circumstances, our injuries and their causes differ widely. Each subsequent time that I speak, I meet at least one person on the panel that I have met previously. The format involves speaking individually for about 15 minutes, followed by a group question and answer period with the students. Our talks focus on our cause of injury, course of hospital stays, if any, and our rehabilitation with primary emphasis on speech-language and cognitive therapy after TBI. I have to refer to my previous invitation from my emails in order to obtain the appropriate wording to describe the format. Even though the format always remains the same. Thinking spontaneously from my head is still difficult. My mind draws a long blank. I have to refer to my or others' written words. We also speak about the good and the not-so-good components of being a participant in TBI therapy.

My first speech is quite an experience. The engagement is a first for a number of reasons for me: public speaking since the crash, talking about my brain injury to a group of people, educating future professionals in the brain injury field and meeting and hearing others with traumatic brain injuries. I am considered the newly injured on this panel in the fifth year of my recovery. For the first time, I am hearing first-hand stories of brain injury and their recovery paths. It is awesome to meet other people like myself in a new community where I finally feel I belong! They are all very functional. I have not met other high-functioning TBI survivors. Functional levels vary widely with TBI survivors. It is exciting but a bit disconcerting as I am face-to-face with mortality – seeing the truth of the possibility that I might not recover to my definition of what recovery means.

From my journal on 2–16–12, the day after my first speech:

> *feeling wowed at meeting and hearing four other TBI survivors talk about similar deficits, things I do, do not do, and am trying to do, all at different levels. Problem – I listened as long as I could but then became overwhelmed with so much information that sounds like noise or static going on. I just could not take in any more information on my mental clipboard. And we were only on panelist 2, I was panelist 4. I was trying to keep my information in the forefront, keep it together, rehearsing in my head and I tried hard to*

know what each was talking about. Scary – information overload.
I now learn of another skill I need to develop further – to hold my
information in my head while listening to another – long enough
to have a conversation. I gain optimism from hearing their stories.

For my part, though, my first speech feels disastrous, although my
journal entry does not dwell on it. From my journal on 2–18–12:

Rick – putting someone at ease – bringing back to subject, and
most importantly making us feel [good about] ourselves – is the
most important thing for an impending therapist. At this speech I
was very nervous – I wrote cryptic notes in large print I could not
read unless I [put it up] to my nose. I brought [a copy for] Rick –
forgot to give it.

I bring a *Rick list*, or itinerary, with me for my speech and a copy to
give to Rick in case I forget my words or freeze. I am disorganized
in my head. I get the papers out but forget to give Rick his copy. I
start my speech, which I cannot read even though it is in large print,
and I hold it close. It is written cryptically, as Rick calls it, in bullet points. I did not flush out the sentences. I finish in about three
minutes. I cannot remember anything else. Rick saves me by asking
questions that prod me along for my time period of 15 whole long
minutes. I develop a new strategy for trying to remember or cue
myself for each succeeding presentation. I have not mastered it yet.
In my most recent speech, in the summer of 2015, I developed a
method where I wrote on cue cards and found a large magnifier on
my iPad. It magnified the cards I held at a reasonable distance so
as to not block my face with the iPad. My growth from preparation
is vast with each experience. My delivery improves. This boosts my
self-esteem, optimism and locus of control, though I am still way
out of my comfort zone.

I feel that I receive even more than I give in these presentations,
which fosters more post-traumatic growth. I am reaching out and
relating to others in innumerable ways. I am learning better coping
techniques, more positive reframing and self-acceptance from the
other panelists. Feeling more open to change as I reflect, I feel even
more of a spiritual shift in my beliefs and experience. I am becoming
more grounded and less disconnected. I have lived by the mantra
that there is always someone else worse off than me, so don't sweat
my load to bear. In this TBI experience, there is such a wide variety
of everlasting symptoms and disabilities to deal with. It is another

way of life. Over this period of time, I see others manage and endure daily activities in spite of their TBI changes and challenges. It is a new way of life for me, and how one lives it is up to our own selves. I am beginning to embrace myself for who I am now, although I still do not embrace having had the TBI. My recovery still has a long way to go for me to consider myself productive or even a viable member of society again, but I experience a measurable shift.

The Support Group

Toward the end of this fifth year, I endeavor with another type of social outreach. Branching out socially, I am now experiencing some relief from the burden of isolation, loneliness and shame. In particular, I am doing this through self-empowerment with the assist from similar others. They understand what the TBI culture and cognitive disability are all about. I investigate a support group for survivors of TBI, and I learn more about my own vulnerabilities. On the first day, I enter a large meeting with people of all levels of TBI: mild, moderate and severe. People's independence levels are diverse. It is a large, crowded room. I feel uncomfortable as even the space around the table seems massive. There are ten of us seated at each large, round table. With my poor vision, it is difficult to see anyone close enough to talk with. And the volume of everyone talking at once is remarkable. I feel lost in this huge crowd. I wonder, does the decibel of the noise bother anyone else to the extent it does me? A speaker is here with an educational film to watch. Amid all of the distractions, I am unable to pay enough attention to benefit from it. I leave feeling dismayed, having failed to make a connection with anyone.

Months later, I go to a smaller group where I am told that a number of group members are at a similar functioning level as me. As in any culture of differences, and not having socialized with people with a TBI, my prejudice or fear of the unknown catches me briefly by surprise. This shocks me to realize it exists in me. I feel trepidation. I do not know what to expect. Will it be a room filled with mes – not comprehending, fatiguing and forgetful, or worse? I am relieved as I am escorted to a squarely arranged set of tables with lovely people all facing each other. They are not as TBIs, but as friendly men and women who all have the same troubles. Fatigue is a number one factor, especially for trying to get there mid-morning – for all of us. Most are not employable because we are on different schedules, needing to rest several times a day and our brains do not function as they used to – speed and processing of information. Although the camaraderie is awesome, I can only attend about seven sessions. The wheelchair lift keeps breaking down in the building. This leaves me with no way to get up to the support group room, which is in a church, an hour and twenty minutes away from my home. I can see the benefits of being in a culture where I feel I belong. I do attend a Christmas party and conference with the group. I try to keep in touch with the facilitator. There is not another group closer to my home. This group motto is "providing support and information, prompting continued rehabilitation, for survivors of acquired brain injuries who are striving to thrive while struggling with cognitive difficulties." Wow! But my social outreach is short-lived.

Gender and the Culture of TBI and PTSD

Feeling my womanhood in the support group for the first time in years, I do further research. I find that leading to marginalization within both women and disability communities is the nature of TBI and the invisibility of cognitive disabilities. I find that women following TBI are particularly vulnerable to psychosocial consequences. They include: disempowerment, isolation, abuse, being less likely to have a career and less likely to have a caregiver. Further, male TBI survivors receive more vocational services and are less likely than women to have such services prematurely terminated, as I did. Arising after brain injury for women are post-morbid emotional themes including: fear of failure, helplessness, powerlessness and humiliation. I identify other themes encompassing loss of dignity, competence, identity and control. Love, fear of future issues of womanhood, sense of mortality, sexual feelings and financial concerns are also among these themes.

I find, too, through research that female TBI survivors are isolated from mainstream support networks and social activities as well as dating opportunities. They are often unemployed, living alone and have few friends. The common problems of transportation, if the TBI results in visual or mobility impairment, and social stigma are significant isolating factors. Investigators find many women report that their slow cognitive processing, communication deficits and memory deficits add to their frustrations. This causes feelings of sadness and depression. Also substantiated is that women living with invisible disabilities can frequently be shunned by other individuals with disabilities. This may leave women behind or on the sidelines within their disability and disabled women communities. It leads to denial of the support that groups can offer. I find there is very little research specific to women with a TBI.

Previous to my TBI, I already had both a visual and mobility impairment, leaving me transportation dependent. I am not employed at this point and still am unable to drive. I lost access to some pre-injury friends and have been too self-conscious about my TBI to make new ones. After losing my identity, for which I took much pride, I wonder how will I regain my self-esteem? How will I recoup a sense of belonging to the world? In my research, I am finding that getting the right emotional support is critical, which researchers assert can be difficult to locate. This is crucial for dismantling the barriers of social alienation that accompany TBI for women. Despite this, I feel ready to complete and end my work with Ellie, my therapist. She has been a most special person for whom I feel a debt of gratitude, as she has truly been a lifesaver. We have become lifelong friends.

18 In the Right Lane
Moving Forward

The Next Level

In the sixth year post-brain injury (2013), I advance to Level IX on the Rancho Los Amigos scale (RLAS), which is marked as:

> **purposeful, appropriate,** needing standby assistance on request. The patient is able to shift between tasks for two hours. Requires some assistance to adjust to life demands. Emotional and behavioral issues may be of concern.
>
> (Hagen et al., 1972, para 9)

My memory loss continues to lead a huge change in my everyday life. This is especially true for communication and understanding, as it does for many with TBI. "Memory is a vehicle to connect the present to the past," states autobiographer and autoethnographer Chang (2008, p. 84). Working on memory is one of my major goals. It is very difficult to research with little access to memories and a small mental clipboard. Mine is continuing to grow. A lot of my memories are likened to unfocused snapshots with many missing. It is hard, too, to hold a lot of information in my brain *and* try to manipulate it. I have been more able to evaluate my circumstances in retrospect, as I am now gaining self-awareness. I believe I am achieving exponential growth in this timeframe. It is visible through the continued writing of my dissertation, my language and cognitive exercises and as I reread my journals and textual records coupled with self-awareness. I still perceive myself as damaged, and I still live in a dichotomy of black or white.

My cognitive capabilities are improving through the process of writing. I am now practicing self-reflection, as I am holding multiple

DOI: 10.4324/9781003428510-23

thoughts in a step. I am learning to think critically again, albeit slowly. I have a passion for my work again, especially since I have come so far through my doctorate program. I am finally ready to get back to my doctoral work. Conversations with Rick affirm a measurement of my improvement and readiness for academic work. Rick states his observation of tremendous growth in me to the point where he believes I can take on the rigors of academia with support. His opinion is paramount to me as he has been conservative with his opinion regarding my ability.

My impact of awareness is increasing in this sixth year post-TBI. I gain a good coping range after my spiritual renewal that entails emotion-focused and problem-focused strategies. I am becoming more optimistic that there is a brighter light somewhere on this path I am trekking. I engage in religious and spiritual coping, seek out social support and continue reappraisal coping. This year is about self-discovery.

I find I am appreciating the value of my life, that it is worth living, though I have not figured out the meaning of my crash. It is still unfathomable. While reappraising the meaning of my car crash, I wrote in my journal on 1–12–13:

> *After my first accident I did find meaning resulting in my advocacy for people with disabilities. I developed new interests – took advantage of new opportunities that I would otherwise not have had. I found meaning in my drastically changed life – found a new purpose- lost faith for a while – went through a reorganization of my spiritual self and came out with a strengthened more meaningful spirituality . . .*

On 1–17–13 I wrote:

> *I guess I went through so many change factors [after the first accident] that I don't embrace it for this accident or rediscovery of myself – again. I gained more resilience after my first car crash recovery, but not enough to have sustained this recovery before now. I can observe this now – I have been clutching tightly to my feeling that I was self-assured and on a great path after such traumata in my life that I believe I was resentful or unwilling to let go, unknowingly. I did have growth posttraumatic after the first.*

I am struggling to use my brain and find meaning.

In February 2013, I discover in my journal reflection that I:

> *lost sense of self-reliance – difficult because I was such a strong person pre-car crash and brain injury – I lost the schema of my persona – wasn't able to handle difficulties and didn't realize I had them for long time – I have been so vulnerable for so long and I despise the way it feels. I have to accept the way things worked out or are working out in order to move on with my life.*

Looking Forward

Intentionally looking towards growth in my research, I find that a large quantity of literature over the past 50 years recognizes the negative outcomes that stress and trauma have on individuals. There is prolific literature on depression, anxiety, heart disease and post-traumatic stress disorder, all resulting from trauma and stress. In more recent literature, thoughts are evolving about the idea that stress and trauma can actually be good for people. I personally and professionally would not go quite that far, but I find that beginning to be addressed are "benefit finding," "post-traumatic stress," and "stress-related growth," for which I do agree.

I found that the causes of PTG (post-traumatic growth) are vast, with reported benefits falling into three categories. They are: (1) feeling stronger and revealing previously unknown hidden strengths and abilities. These positively change self-concept and confidence to face new encounters; (2) strengthening good relationships, which reflects a finding of who their true friends are after experiencing the trauma; and (3) philosophies and priorities are altered to prioritize relationships and living for the moment. There is consistency in the literature regarding the benefits. One researcher describes the same type of benefits as emotional growth, closer family relationships and a better perspective on life. These benefits reflect my evolving outlook during this period.

As I am more able to reflect, I find I also have an openness to new experiences. My emotions are more stable. I have improved my optimism and self-esteem. These are personality factors that are associated with greater post-traumatic growth. My coping techniques continue to involve seeking social support, acceptance, turning to religion and more positive reframing. Optimism is defined as the general expectancy on self-report by survivors for good things to happen compared to bad things. I am starting to view the world this way again instead of the constant feeling of impending doom. I also have a propensity for interest in new situations, new experiences and new ideas, which implies openness.

Community Integration

Having a renewed appreciation of life and feeling more self-reliant, I begin to connect myself socially through group membership, common experiences and personal contact. I do this by opening myself to new possibilities, and hence PTG. I have some involvement with the TBI support group. I receive mailings of happenings monthly. I am following their interests by group email, although I do not often have much to add. I attend a few special meetings when held outside of the church. I continue to perform social actions, speaking again on a panel of speakers with the common experience of a TBI and rehabilitation. These engagements are at Boston University in the spring and summer semesters of 2013.

I connect with several other panelists and am keeping in personal contact with one. This is a big step for me as I still find talking on the phone difficult. Christy, one of the panelists, does as well. I keep phone calls short before I totally fatigue and lose the conversation. I have continued troubles with memory, the organization and delivery of my speeches and fatigue. I make more progress each time (!), though, and I am learning more about myself. I am discovering that I *am* stronger than I thought I was with the evolution of each new speech. I focus on elaborating a bit more each time and am more aware of the present of my story. I am gaining more life satisfaction as I compare my TBI rehabilitation with those on the panel. I am learning more boundaries for my strengths and my limitations.

I am attending my first conference and becoming a member of the Brain Injury Association of Massachusetts (BIA-MA) as a survivor in February 2013. I find that BIA-MA is a non-profit organization that provides support to brain injury survivors and their families. They offer programs to prevent brain injuries and educate the public on the risks and impact of brain injury. They advocate for legislation and funding for services. The conference has workshops for survivors, their families and professionals, offering continuing education credits for appropriate professionals. My professional license, an LMHC (Licensed Mental Health Counselor), which I have managed to keep current, is approved for these credits. As a survivor, I am given strategies for how to get through the conference. This includes quiet rooms separated for brain injury survivors who need to take a break from overstimulation. It is overwhelming, but I am running into people I know from the support group, Spaulding Rehabilitation Hospital and a colleague who is an LMHC. I am relating to people on different levels: as a fellow survivor, as a friend, my former patient/client and a colleague. I feel multidimensional for the first time in years!

I continue to be the Chairperson for the Wilmington Commission on Disability, for which I keep a fairly low profile. In August 2013, my Town Manager appoints me to serve as a member of the Open Space and Recreation Commission. As per the Americans with Disabilities Act (ADA) of 1990, the town does not discriminate on the basis of disability, and there has to be accountability. This pertains to program applicants, participants, members of the general public, employees, job applicants and others who are entitled to participate in and benefit from all town programs, activities and services without regard to disability. I am looking at facilities under the jurisdiction of the conservation commission and several other outside properties not owned by the conservation commission. They are important recreational assets to the town, requiring assessment for compliance with regards to accessibility.

An example property is the Town Beach, fishing pier and Baby Beach. The use level is high. Activities enabled are swimming, picnicking, sunbathing, playing in the sand and on the playground, boating, fishing and nature observation. I am assessing the Town Beach parking lot, bathhouse changing rooms and family toilets for handicapped accessibility under the law. I find there is a paved, level walkway that connects the handicapped-accessible fishing pier to the gravel portion of the beach parking lot, which is compliant. For Baby Beach, users walk to the beach. I find, however, that the sidewalks are on the opposite side of the street. For a transition plan, improvements need to include connecting the sidewalk from one side to the other. As well, my recommendations are a textured wheelchair access walkway on the beach, a surf chair, which is a wheelchair that can roll over sand and universal picnic tables that accommodate all, including wider space and height appropriate for a wheelchair, all of which I locate. Other access issues include the need for signage and tactile projection warnings for people with sight impairments. This requires hours of work and intense concentration from me, but it is personally rewarding.

My participation is slow-going, especially as I try to read and understand plans and requirements. I have to reread sentences and paragraphs of specifications, laws and materials several times each in order to understand the information, which was rote for me pre-injury. I am now able to appreciate the reward of meeting people who know me from where I am now, with no expectations to a standard for which I am no longer capable. I am not spontaneous during the commission meetings. I have to actually go home and go through my notes before I can think clearly enough to formulate a thought and make a decision. I explain my TBI sequelae in brief to some of the commissioners as my interaction is noticeably quiet. I am, however, able to do work from home between our infrequent meetings.

My writing for my dissertation is moving along and greatly improving. In September 2013, I join a writing group once a month with three other PhD candidates and my lovely doctoral committee Chairperson, Julia. Julia is on each of our committees. We read pieces of each other's work that we are struggling with and help flesh them out for more clarity. It is rewarding and stimulating to hear each other's exciting work, as we all are adding new information to our fields. There is a real sense of great fellowship.

Trek Four

Ultimately Blossoming in the Sun: Paving a Way

Years 7 and Beyond Post-TBI: Toward New Growth: Hope

19 Opening Passageways

Discovering Insight, Value and Growth

In this seventh year (2014) and beyond, I progress to Level X on the Rancho Los Amigos Recovery scale (RLAS) marked as:

> **purposeful, appropriate,** where needs are seen as modified independent. The patient is goal-directed, handling multiple tasks and independently using assistive strategies. Prone to breaks in attention and may require additional time to complete tasks. These levels are guidelines and patients go back and forth between stages.
> (Hagen et al., 1972, para 10)

This above description is an example of some of my days. Multitasking skills are still quite difficult. In this timeframe, I gain hope and acceptance. This period is stimulating for me. I find it easier to reflect and interpret in spite of my traumatic brain injury. Of special note is that a new medication for cognition is now available, specifically for memory. Most prominent trials have been done with people with moderate to severe Alzheimer's Disease. I have been following the protocol of another such medication, Aricept, also prescribed predominantly for Alzheimer's Disease. I cannot wholly vouch for it, though. In March 2014, I start taking the new medication, Namenda, in conjunction with the Aricept twice a day. It is helping immensely! My memory is stronger. I have better focus and concentration for longer periods of time. My memory capacity is increased. My attention and retention noticeably grow so much that my doctor doubles the dose in June 2014.

From my journal 8–13–14:

> *I have been clearer in my writing and what I want to say. I feel more direct rather than dancing around a subject. I can hold several thoughts and try to manipulate them. I feel like I am breaking*

DOI: 10.4324/9781003428510-25

out of captivity. It is not a wonder drug. Taken with my other medication and still working hard at my skills and strategies I am making positive strides. I can think a bit – more – again – far more than my dark cloak and spacey days, which I still have occasionally. My brain is exhausted from all of this discovery and jubilance. Things are looking up! I still have to pace myself and follow my other brain strategies.

I develop insight. From my journal 8–25–14:

Through this research process – autoethnography – I have developed more insight and information about traumatic brain injury and posttraumatic stress that I am having growth myself. This has been remarkable for me. I had been plagued with anxiety and depression. Learning about TBI and how to improve my skills, learning compensatory skills and – learned how and where I could work on recovery, and from the brain injury workbook, I have made large strides toward posttraumatic growth after TBI and PTSD. I will never be the same, but I have/am learning to live with the "me" now, and strive for the best. I have a "new normal." It is a combination of actually getting better, forgetting how it used to be, and adapting to changes around me and how I now do things. I stopped doing certain things because it is just not possible or is just not that important for me to spend that much energy on.

Valuing My Life

From my journal (8–27–14):

my observation today is that I feel my sense of purpose is still developing. I am attaining a growing sense of personal meaning. I am discovering that I need to take an even greater stock of my life and realize that which affects my everyday living. I am back to basics with my head out of the fog. I do feel my life satisfaction is growing. I am still resolute on finishing this essential dissertation, and am seeing possibilities for its use in my near future. My number of activities has increased, starting with working more in my rose garden with twelve bushes. I remain the chairperson for the Commission on Disability and continue my appointment to the Open Space and Recreations Commission. Both meet infrequently. It's nice to be able to think for a minute of something and someone else.

Since my injury, I have also increased my relationships and social supports. I am closer to family members. I have two new friendships with women who also have TBI's and are high functioning. At this time, I now observe that I do have an affirmation of spiritual values and my religious faith.

Contemplation in my journal (8–29–14):

As I center myself this night, I am now just starting to see the new direction for my life. With outstretched arms, reclined somewhat in my power wheelchair, I feel my renewed appreciation for each day of my valued life. It travels from my head, down into my forehead, streams through my face, branches out down my arms, travelling all the way through to my fingertips. It surges into my torso and spreads through all of my body. With my eyes closed I hear the classical music from Bolero playing down the hall. There is a quietness and stillness in this room. The aroma of marinara sauce simmering in the kitchen fills my nostrils and my stomach faintly rumbles. I am contemplating that we are here on earth for a relatively short time, and grasping for the meaning of this particular day. I am at peace in this moment.

The next evening, (8–30–14) in my journal:

In this special place, each night I put into words a gratitude list of what I am grateful for this day – people, places and things, whatever positive happened this day. Struggling in the beginning has been difficult to name two – grown the list to minimum of five each night. For instance: I am grateful I am even able to do this coping skill. I am grateful for my children and family members, for Jay, for the register clerk who made a joke which made me smile, and for my roses. I am also reminded that I am incredibly grateful for Marquis [my service dog] for his great love and assistance. Today he got me the phone from the cradle on the kitchen counter, opened the refrigerator and got my water bottle out, brought it to me, picked up the mail I dropped, shut the back door when he came in (and got a special treat), picked up my pen twice, got me a pillow off the couch and brought it to me, and stretched his front paws up to my shoulders for a hug. He also pulled my towel off the rack and brought it to me in the shower. Doing such a grateful list is a fine exercise to stretch my brain at the end of each day.

In this year, 2014, I continue to see Rick for cognitive therapy every two to three weeks, where we work on my writing and thinking skills, cognitive strategies and aspects of my dissertation. I attend assistive technology therapy for two long periods beginning in March 2014 and August 2014, relearning the capabilities of my iPad and how to transcribe from my tape recorder on the iPad. I also work on remembering how to use Dragon Naturally Speaking. These are all tools I use to write my dissertation. I have been using them, but in turn, forgot almost completely after a short term of non-use. This is a revolving problem for me in utilizing high and low assistive technology. It takes many repetitions and many organized notes to become memorable.

Physically, my shoulder, neck and head are still in pain. I continue to have a prolonged loss of range of motion with my right shoulder, arm and pectoral muscles. I am considering surgery, as my doctor feels confident it will help me. I want to finish writing my dissertation first. It will require my arm to be in a sling for six to eight weeks, which will interfere with my writing and care for myself. At this point, I think it is just permanent. Wheeling my manual wheelchair is not possible on a permanent basis since the day of the second car crash. I am managing my fatigue by pacing myself and taking necessary breaks before and after so that I can make accomplishments daily. All of my efforts are in the writing of my dissertation. I am working in two-hour sprints through the day and night, seven days a week. It takes an enormous amount of effort after I know what I want to write to actually formulate and write each sentence. I literally fall asleep for a time after each writing period.

The struggle to understand my traumata eventually strengthens my religious beliefs. It further helps me find a way to intimacy and increases my sense of control. Involved are alterations to my basic assumptions. Recognizing meaning in the center of my trauma and its aftermath, finally creating momentum, is leading to a new philosophy of life. I perceive spiritual and relational changes, which allow my experiences of coping strategies to have a greater effect in this area of my life. I am developing more personal strength physically, spiritually and emotionally, and am becoming open to new possibilities, which allows my spiritual growth. Difficulty in my capabilities in learning and benefiting from this life experience, after having done so a number of times previously, is contemplated. Benefits, I am finding, are potential elements of my continued developing wisdom. It is captured in this anonymous insightful quote that I have posted on my refrigerator for many years, "we cannot direct the wind, but we can adjust the sails."

Developing Wisdom

I am reconstructing and building up my perception of self, others and the meaning of events. This is possible through reflection in this timeframe and from my experience with the individuals in the support group, my associate panel speakers, Claudia Osborn (1998) and my language-cognitive therapy. My willingness to accept help leads to more emotional expressiveness. I have closer family relationships and a deepening of relationships with others who have suffered a TBI. I am finding what is changeable and what is not by circumstances and acceptance. I have an awareness, and I am ready to face new possibilities, which is another factor of PTG. I do not feel I am able to do better things with my life, but I feel now that I am better able to do things in and with my life post-trauma.

In reflection, I have come to realize that if someone is totally healed, and all the scars are eliminated from what took place in the experience, the individual is still changed because going through the experience alone changes us. Developing an appreciation of what one has or has lost will change one's life view forever. In this vision, there is no going back to the "old" you. It is my position that a traumatic experience is exponentially greater and the losses much more extreme, especially the loss of self physically, emotionally and spiritually. I will never have my life back as I knew it. No one can. And that is now okay.

Life, I find, is all about changes and transitions. Change is inevitable. I have several pearls of wisdom that help describe my new outlook: "A bridge of silver wings stretches from the dead ashes of an unforgiving nightmare to the jeweled vision of a life started anew" (Aberjhani, 2010, p. 54), which decisively describes my poetic journey. And, "Healing doesn't mean the damage never existed. It means the damage no longer controls our lives" (rawforbeauty. com). Through it all, I have learned that "We acquire the strength we have overcome" (Ralph Waldo Emerson, motivatingquotes.com/ strength/html). I have, too, found that we cannot hurry growth.

During an office visit in September 2014, while reviewing my progress, Dr. T., my specialist for TBI and PTSD informs me that I am a success story and a role model! The reason is my continuing recovery from TBI and PTSD. He notes as well my progress and tenacity on my dissertation, which I am writing daily. I am able to do analysis and interpretation, a huge accomplishment for my brain. Dr. T. credits my success, too, for my participation and success on the speaker panel at Boston University, which is more fluent this year. He has me take a moment to reflect upon where I am and from where I have come. I am only 65% of what I used to be, with many other changes in deficits and benefits. I continue with my daily struggles.

Community Integration

My community integration expands in 2014 and 2015. Realizing that I have lots of room for recovery and improvement, and at the suggestion of my doctoral committee, I try to flex my brain capacity by taking a writing course at the Cambridge Center for Adult Education. In March 2014, I enroll in an eight-week course entitled *Writing from your experience,* a writing workshop. I find it wonderfully helpful in so many ways. I am out in the community and sitting in a room with seven other adults. Not knowing my circumstances, I am accepted for who I am now. I feel extremely vulnerable, but I know that others feel vulnerable, too, since several of us read what we write each week. Actually, I am terrified and don't feel worthy to be here. I am writing, but am I really a writer again?

I increase my ability to pay more attention to others and to hold more information in my head. I push myself to speak, and as I read out loud, I hope my thoughts are in a coherent piece of writing. I listen through my earplug as the speech processor on my computer reads a line. I then repeat what I hear and try to keep an even flow as I listen to the next sentence. I stammer through it. I compel myself to read out loud on three occasions, each time a bit less than one page. This is the capacity of my writing. I appreciate the feedback, and I grow my writing skills. By the end of the course, I am no longer feeling myself as unequal. I relate well with everyone. The group does find out about my traumatic brain injury due to the content of my writing. I am using pieces for my dissertation. I begin to open my writing experiences with fluency. I discover and work on the ability to change my texts by moving bits, rewriting and discarding content. I gain a feeling of mounting control over more than writing a sentence, but also control over the shape, texture and energy of a sentence. I am inspired.

Successful in many ways, I know I can benefit even more. I brace myself, as I have lots of apprehension. I make the call to sign up for another eight-week course in June 2014: *Getting personal: a memoir and essay workshop*. I open myself to the elements again. There are 11 students around a very large rectangle of connected tables. It feels more like 20 people, maybe because we are so spread out. About halfway through the first session, I begin to relax a bit. In this workshop, we again write every week, and everyone reads their stories aloud each session. In my stories, I write deeper, using material for my dissertation. I gain knowledge by concentrating on ways to frame my memories, tighten focus and clarify feelings and opinions. I actually have to think and formulate opinions, which is still a sluggish process for me. I extend my thinking outside my box. I gain greatly from each and every classmate and our freelance writer/teacher. Through their feedback, my meager feedback to them, writing, sharing and holding our intimate stories, I grow. My dissertation writing is budding.

In September 2014, feeling more familiar with the process, I once more take an eight-week course: *Living stories*, a workshop for beginner and advanced writers. My writing and flow are enhanced. I learn more about the texture of the story and where I am in relation to what I am writing. Strategies to overcome persistent difficulties in writing, taught through exercises, take me away from my topic. Writing creatively and on different subject matters sparks new life and ideas into my dissertation writing. I truly enjoy this session. My ways of relating, sense of self and changing philosophy of life are ever-increasing.

Social Actions

During this timeframe, I continue with my daily struggles. That is my new way of life. I am adjusting. Nonetheless, I venture out to participate in a few social actions. In 2014, I sign up to become an Ambassador for the Brain Injury Association of Massachusetts (BIA-MA) to support their cause for their Brain Injury Affects Campaign. BIA-MA collaborates with the Massachusetts Rehabilitation Commission, the Department of Public Health and the Veterans Administration. As an ambassador, I am to represent BIA-MA and convey their powerful message to civic and community groups about brain injury through my personal story. Working with an Advocacy Associate through an interview technique, we are able to encapsulate my brain injury story into one and a half pages. Involved is what happened to me and how it has affected my life. Through my unique experience, I can help change the lives of others and myself and provide hope. Saying what is on my mind can be a petition for change. I will also present information on the programs and services of BIA-MA. They are committed to educating the public about brain injury and empowering survivors and their families to live their fullest lives possible. BIA-MA advocates for improved services for survivors and proactively supports legislation to prevent brain injury.

While my endeavor is limited, I am also asked to become an Advocate, which connects my past with my present. I contact my State Representative and State Senator to request their support on relevant Bills regarding continued brain injury services and services for eligible brain injury survivors. There are currently 3,000 people with a TBI on a waiting list for services in Massachusetts. One such line item is to urge the designation of 100% of the collections received by the courts from DUI and DWI Violations to go into the HITS Fund to support community-based brain injury services. This will help preserve services at no cost to the State. The aim is to urge legislators to designate the funds for increased residential services, day programs, a multi-service center and case management services to begin to meet the needs of the 3,000 people on the waiting list. Elected officials maintain that the most effective advocacy is from constituents, especially from those with a personal moving story. In this case, it is about brain injury and the life-changing effect of state-supported services. In my case, I have been fortunate to have had case management.

In 2015, BIA-MA is advocating at the State House for the passage of the joint State and House bill S.485/H.843, an Act Relative to Cognitive Rehabilitation. The joint bill will require private insurance companies to cover post-acute cognitive rehabilitation for individuals with acquired and traumatic brain injury. This, again, is at no cost to the State. BIA-MA put a call out for written testimonials from survivors and their families. They want to know how survivors are having trouble attaining services or how services are helping. I take my action one step further. On 11–5–15, I testify at the hearing of the Joint Committee on Financial Services at the State House, a committee of 18, although not all are present. The testimonial has to be succinct and no longer than three minutes. Challenging my communication abilities, I am able to contain my complete testimonial to one page. At a heavy wooden desk with a microphone in the middle, I sit before the Joint Committee, Marquis by my side, and make my address. I share my experience of post-acute cognitive rehabilitation services and the denial from my healthcare insurance to continue, even though I was still making progress. I articulate my continuance as a private payer and the progress and accomplishments I have made. I speak about returning to the writing of my dissertation and my reinstatement to my PhD program. This speech is a success!

I complete a third supplemental action as I visit my State Senator and Representative to urge them to support the bill. Representative James Miceli, still in office, greets me with open arms. We have worked very closely on disability advocacy and civil rights for many, many years, beginning in the 1980s before people with disabilities were visible to the public. We know each other on a personal level. We have fought actively side by side. Jim has spoken at numerous events sponsored by my social and political groups, including the one-year anniversary of our first successful integrated disability social center that integrated people with cross disabilities (not common at that time) and non-disabled people. Happening in 1988, I was president of the Wilmington Committee for Citizens with Disabilities (WCCD), a non-profit organization for the betterment of people with disabilities. We received a citation from Governor Dukakis that reads, "Which is deserving of recognition by all the citizens of Massachusetts." Also offered by Representative Miceli in 1988, we received a citation from the House of Representatives, signed by then Speaker of the House George Keverian.

Representative Jim listens to me and reads my testimonial. I have not been in touch with Jim since shortly after my car crash in 2007. As I share and update my life history, I bring about awareness of brain injury. In spite of my tremendous efforts in recovery, Jim witnesses instantly my changes due to the TBI. He remarks about my speaking, writing and demeanor. Consequently, he recognizes this issue as paramount, and he demonstrates support for the bill. As well, Jim offers me support in any other way I may need. This brings full circle a major facet of my life.

During this timeframe of 2014 and beyond, I also develop and maintain friendships with three of the women I have met on the Boston University speaking panels. We all have TBIs. We all work hard to preserve our friendships. We share the difficulties of fatigue, remembering, initiating and having a diminished memory capacity for retention and word retrieval. We clearly understand each other when we get together. It is actually fun and a relief to be around others where we can just be ourselves. We understand each other's daily grind and method of accomplishing tasks. We are genuinely happy for each other's accomplishments, tiny and big. Most of our tiny accomplishments require mammoth efforts. We share the same adjustment to our cultural standards and challenges. And, too, we share our adjustment to our changed language and way of thinking, perceiving, evaluating and behaving. I haven't had fun in my language since before the car crash in 2007.

20 Trail Blazing onto a Steady Path

Blossoming into Disability Culture

In 2015, I feel I am back on sturdy ground. I still see Rick approximately every three weeks. Rick's Speech-Language Pathology Daily Note of 11–6–15 provides an example of what we are currently working on. It is also about the progress I am making in my daily life. I have a daily life with happenings beyond survival and trying to write a sentence – Yeah! I am able to present what I have been doing over the past three weeks, which Rick helps me to organize. He then assists me in enunciating what I want to work on in today's session. I take more control over the session today rather than having Rick lead. Rick's note states that our session focus is on: written expression, attention and organization. Rick's succinct note, much fuller than my brief notes, reveals:

> Patient arrives without computer today so does not take notes on this session. Patient states she testified yesterday at the State House regarding bill on cognitive rehabilitation. She presented one page of text. She was nervous initially but after seeing others she states she relaxed and did well. She notes strategies of using very large font to compensate for severe visual impairment, double spaced, with bullet points at beginning of lines. She has continued to take writing course through Cambridge Adult Ed and shares a new poem. Her writing has improved dramatically over this year. From Audio Memo files recorded in previous session, clinician was commenting on aspect of patient's response to the book about recovery from TBI, Over My Head, and patient requested that this be recorded. Patient will attempt to integrate this information into her thesis. Patient notes she had positive meeting with one of her thesis advisors. One of the recommendations is that patient improve the links in between sections of her manuscript. Clinician discussed research that finds written narrative by TBI patient is weak in "cohesive ties"

DOI: 10.4324/9781003428510-26

between segments. Patient will bring in section of manuscript next visit and we will address use of language to summarize and convey transitions to the next theme.

Of note patient shows overall increased sustained attention and increased working memory for auditory information.

Writing Grief

With my writing beginning to flourish and my socializing broadening, I look at the 2015 CCAE course catalog for writing under my Optilec, my magnification reading machine. I find the perfect workshop. It is an eight-week course entitled *The poetry of grief and trauma, advanced poetry workshop.* The workshop seems to encapsulate my trauma experiences and innate poetry writing. I find I am able to explore difficult subject matter in poetry without the risk of drowning in it. Writing a poem, to me, is a way to assemble a little bit of order in the midst of the chaos of trauma. My expressiveness is dramatically improved and my recovery boosted. In this course, I explore my circumstances through different forms of poetry. I take this course in the summer semester. Due to the chemistry and success of our group, all but one of us take the course again in Fall 2015 with the same instructor. We continue. We are all advanced poetry writers who take our work seriously but are vulnerable with our subject matter. We all give honest and astoundingly useful feedback as we help each other rework our pieces. I know I am back to being a writer! On 8–5–15, I pen:

The Taken

What did I take?

You shook from me a piece of my brain
You took from me my thinking mind
You took my speed and ability to process information
You took my dignity and pride
You took my ability to remember what happened
You took my memory, short and sometimes long term, I can't
remember
You took from me my words
You took my ability to read and write
You took my ability to pay attention and comprehend
You took my sense of humor
You took my agility
You took from me my spirit, but I took it back

Why did I take – again?

You said I am strong enough to handle it
You said so I may help others with the same afflictions
You said because my mind was always thinking
Until I could hardly remember

How did I take it?

By shaking my head fiercely forward and backward
By disconnecting my memories
By slowing my thought processes
You said I let my guard down

Where did I take you?

Onto the long and fuzzy highway, you took me
Under the dark cloak of the night you took me
Into the foggy never-land where words cannot reach you
    took me
Under the stands of cheering fans at Fenway loud and loud you
    took me
Over the moon with the dog and the spoon you took me
Feeling the thick fog roll in as the stamina rolled out you
    took me

Who did I take you from?

You took me from my children
You took me from my family members
You took me from my colleagues
You took me from my community
You took me from my cultures
You took me from my best friend
You took me from myself

When did I take you?

You seized me when I was not looking
You seized me when I was admiring nature's beauty
You seized me when I was in the time of my life
You seized me when my sister was dying

What did I give you?

You gave me angst
You gave me hopelessness
You gave me fatigue
You gave me loneliness
But my endurance and will held strong
Turned into new self-perception
Turned into new relationships
Turned into new philosophy of life

I give me growth after all that has been taken.

In another poem, I am finally able to write my story succinctly:

Life-changing Crash

With spring in full swing on a warm, sunny day
Flourishing flowering trees in the breeze sway
Magnolias, dogwoods, and roses scent a way
Into open car windows this sixth day in May.

Onto the highway the pair southbound hopped
Travelling with speed to the mall they would shop
On the ramp of the interchange traffic stopped
Across the back seat her service dog flopped.

Suddenly thrust forward her head hit the dash
Seatbelt jerked violently, the headrest she smashed
Accelerate-decelerate forced her brain to thrash
The impact was huge in this life-changing crash.

Rammed by a truck at sixty-five miles an hour
Her wheelchair and trunk pushed in with such power
To the front headrest crushed and devoured
Forced upon car in front, they were overpowered.

Knocked unconscious briefly, rotator cuff torn,
Her neck was sprained deeply, and muscle aches worn
He was jumbled up deeply, muscle spasms adorn
The dog swayed freakily, pinned to headrest, forlorn.

The ambulance came and whisked them to care
The dog had a seizure, he was doing fair
Strapped on a board they continued to stare
CT of the neck, her head injury unaware.

Home they all went, sleep off and on she begot
Waking to same questions, her memory shot
Severe headaches for weeks she suffered a lot.
Word-finding and brain function were all for not.

Grieving for the pain and each and every loss
Of body functions not working, wiped out across
Her head, neck and shoulder, right arm she can't toss
She is down to one limb; the paraplegia is boss.

Horror and helplessness, injured severely
A second time hurt, life fairness – not really
Losing her mind after physical loss clearly
Dazed and confused she tried to know, wearily.

Traumatic brain injury, now lost in a fog
Minutes of clarity let her out of the bog
But her mind held hostage is not easy to jog
Unfathomable fatigue, she drags like a dog.

Onto rehab for speech therapy she went
Language and cognitive skills she also was sent
To learn to read and write, pre-primers were lent
With pages for nursery school children they're meant.

She struggled with fragments and phrases to write
And could not decipher, what a miserable plight
A sentence to remember took all of her might
Taking notes on a paragraph – oh what a fight.

Where will this lead, to her doctorate she hopes,
With long way to go, does she have many hopes?
She met similar others who shared their ropes
She is still rehabbing, but now she copes.

On 10–24–15, I pen a light-hearted poem that exposes my new attitude:

I Shine

Upon a heavenly day
Wind chimes in the air
And yes, I shine
I nurture, cherish, and
care for you
All that you are
   And that you're not
Tranquil,
Hear the wind chime
Hear the wind-chimes
And again, I shine
Drift into my glow.

Years Beyond

I again update the literature review chapter of my dissertation for my areas of interest, especially for TBI and PTG, which I have been doing each year now. My narrative chapter is close to completion. During the past two years, I have been met with serious health and injury-related issues that caused another brief leave of absence from school and a delay in finishing. As many of us do, I have also been caretaking my father, who has been an inspirational and joyful companion, living in my home until he lost his battle with brain cancer and heart disease. My final poem:

My Father's Condition

In the coldness and darkness and still of the night you cried out but only a whisper was heard, "you better make the call." As I watch you struggle to draw breath into your swollen silhouette illuminated in the shadow, your stomach distended, lungs drowning in fluid, I feel the cold blank stare before your eyes roll into your pasty face. I touch you. Your clammy, sweaty body, and your arms so cold, the white hairs on your arm pronounced against your speckled skin, your parched lips part as I hear the torment of your shallow breath. A churning inside me as I witness your struggle, the dog lain by your feet, a whining howl he lets out. The pain and the truth. I am reaching out to you. Can you hear me call? Activity gone. Finally, at the door flashing red and white lights. Rushing in are the paramedics. Oxygen. . . . And more. It is not your time to go.

And then it was, 12–3–16.

I lost a major supportive relationship and true friend.

My road to recovery blazes on. In this time period, I experience my greatest growth. I have regained critical thinking. With it, I began to see myself not only through the lens of my prior experiences but through reflection on those experiences. I realize post-traumatic growth. PTG is a phenomenon of growth in the aftermath of suffering extreme life adversities. These adversities challenge one's core beliefs and worldviews in a way in which one's psychological well-being is positively changed. In the aftermath of trauma, some survivors come to realize that not all goals are attainable. They cannot integrate their new reality into their previous assumptive world. In order to rebuild shattered worldviews, a meaning-making process occurs, resulting in a perception of growth. It is the outcome of trying to cope with trauma and decrease feelings of distress. Leading to a transformed identity, changes can be seen in self-perception, interpersonal relationships and philosophies of life. I found PTG is a paradox wherein losses can generate beneficial and valued gains. Although PTG may not happen for everyone, it happened for me. It happens for about 60% of trauma survivors. I was surprised and amazed as my early efforts and future seemed quite bleak.

There is an assessment tool to measure PTG called the Posttraumatic Growth Inventory (PTGI) developed by Tedeshci & Calhoun in 1996. The domains encompass: factor I, relating to others; factor II, new possibilities; factor III, personal strength; factor IV, spiritual change; and factor V, appreciation of life. Utilizing the self-report statements on this inventory, I analyzed my growth from my journal entry statements. My summary of growth follows.

In the timeframe of Years 1 and 2, I had no post-traumatic growth. In the timeframe of Years 3 and 4, I started demonstrating post-traumatic growth through Factor I. This became visible in relating to others, as I came to know, "I can count on people in times of trouble." I started to "accept needing others," and I also started "putting effort into my relationships." In the timeframe of Years 5 and 6, my growth is seen through Factors I, III, IV and V. In the factor of relating to others, my growth expanded as I developed "a willingness to express my emotions" and continued "putting effort into my relationships." I showed growth through personal strength, as seen by developing "a feeling of self-reliance," discovering "that I am stronger than I thought I was," and in "being able to accept the way that things worked out." With regard to spiritual change, I established that "I have a stronger religious faith" and "a better understanding of spiritual matters." I also showed growth through my new appreciation of life. I fostered an "appreciation for the value of my own life," as well as "appreciating each day."

In the timeframe of Years 7 and Beyond, my post-traumatic growth increased, evidenced through Factors I, II, III and V. In relating to others, I cultivated "a sense of closeness with others," and "I learned a great deal about how wonderful people are." I gained more personal strength as I regained the knowledge that "I can handle difficulties." I grew more of an appreciation of life as I re-established "my priorities about what is important in life." My greatest growth in this timeframe is with the factor of new possibilities, which I did not develop in any other time frame. I was able to "establish a new path for my life" and "develop new interests." I began to "change things which needed changing," and I realized "I am able to do better things with my life."

Disability as a Culture

Society needs to accept that disability is a universal facet of the human experience. At some stage of their lives, disability will affect almost all members. Through birth, accident, natural disaster, illness, war or poverty, anyone can become disabled. This is without regard to age, class, race or gender.

Culture, I found, is the way of life of a group of people: their behaviors, beliefs, values and symbols that they accept. Generally, it is done without thinking. They are passed along by communication and imitation from one generation to the next. Members of the disability culture have shared close and comparable beliefs, values and behaviors. They are learned and shared, however, by members of a group since the majority do not have parents that are disabled. Group membership as disabled allows for quality and control over their own lives and community.

Society has viewed people with disabilities as having a physical or mental problem, who have a dependence on family members and professionals and have a lack of educational, socio-economic, political and cultural skills. They are seen as having a lack of legal protection, hostile attitudes and environments and a loss of worth as a disabled person. Society labels disabled people as pathological and defective and need *fixing* or *curing* in order to adapt to the environment to fit in. Society has portrayed disabled people as victims of circumstance who are worthy only of pity. Compartmentalizing people with disabilities into what is wrong with them and as less than the general population is inappropriate and wrong.

There has been a distinct separate culture for persons who share the inability to work, play or perform an age-appropriate life function because of a physical or mental impairment. An uprising of people with disabilities found their own voices to demonstrate their actual experiences with disability. Issues included common experience, segregation, oppression, tolerance, barriers and then became celebration and unity.

Disability culture is the second phase of the disability movement. It is a mission for collective identity and self-determination. The word *disabled* represents a social identity of awareness and empowerment within the culture. People with disabilities started changing the perception of disability from that of weak and disregarded to strong and valued. Vying to counter oppression, the disability culture challenged the societal norms as a civil rights movement. Laws and civil rights for people with disabilities were fought hard for and won by disability activists and certain politicians. The remedy to oppression was full integration of people with disabilities to guarantee full participation in society. Civil rights were won for people with disabilities, which culminated in the 1990 Americans with Disabilities Act (ADA).

Disabled people are not victims. Disability is not a brave struggle. It is not courage in the face of adversity. It is not a reduction in value to live with a disability than to live without it.

Disability culture is a compilation of new values. It is life-affirming. Since people with disabilities have a shared consciousness, most share a strong bond between them.

Expressing culture in a unified way, people with disabilities communicate their goals, values and identities. Consequently, to the public, it allows them to project a positive image. Presenting a strong image motivates people to want to belong and to be a part of something powerful. Disability culture is the difference between being alone and isolated with a disability that in our society invites discrimination and isolation and being in a community. Through the view of disability culture, disability as a way of life is neither tragic nor devalued.

Core values for people with disabilities differ from those of the general society. They include an acceptance of human vulnerability. They value interdependence over the illusion of independence. They prize self-determination over self-sufficiency. Another value is an acceptance of human differences. Next is a humor to laugh at the most dreadful of circumstances/oppressors. They value not functional separateness but rather personal connection, and not physical autonomy, but human community. Other core values include a value of expansive ways to move through the world. Lastly, a tolerance for the lack of resolution of the randomness and unpredictability of life is valued.

Through the disability cultural movement, people with disabilities have empowered themselves as agents of their own lives. With that empowerment, they changed the archetype of disability to what they determined it should be: culture, rights and pride. This shift of disability asserts that the consequences of differences materialize as celebrations. Society has a lot to gain from the concept that people with disabilities are contributing members of society. The shared experience of disability can be a source of empowerment in fostering personal growth, reconciling with one's disability and may also promote acceptance of human differences.

Disability culture emphasizes a way of living and positive identification with being disabled. Many people, including people with disabilities, do not identify with disability as a culture or a right. They continue to see disability as an impairment. I offer my story to help achieve healing to realize disability is not about shame and humiliation, but about dignity and virtue to gain strength, empowerment and growth. My hope, too, is for people with disabilities to continue their life's journey as worthwhile. I hope that reading/hearing my story will raise awareness of disability identity as a source of pride, not pity. Sharing similar stories of oppression and ridicule, acknowledging humorous anecdotes and witnessing another survivor succeed in recovery may change another's attitude – one struggling with early recovery and feelings of hopelessness.

My actions for change will continue through counseling, advocacy, motivational speaking and continued writing. I am no longer ashamed of my TBI-PTSD and paraplegia. I am proud of who I am, proud of what I have overcome and proud of my disability culture. Being a part of this culture has given me a sense of community, comfort and support that motivates me. I am not alone. I lost a lot of who I was, but now at this stage of my recovery, I am my new normal.

The last thought Rick, my speech therapist, gave to me was:

The most striking aspect of Dee's recovery has been how far she has come from the days when she struggled to hold a two-minute NPR news clip in her memory to now completing her doctoral degree. Her singular will and determination have driven her recovery and reset our equations for what is possible after traumatic brain injury.

(R. Richard Sanders, M.S.CCC, M.T.S. Senior Speech-Language Pathology Clinical Specialist at Spaulding Rehabilitation Hospital in Charlestown, MA)

My final thought is that a beautiful life is not always produced in ideal conditions. I liken my recovery journey to a lotus flower, rising through mud and adversity, petals opening one by one and ultimately blossoming in the sun.

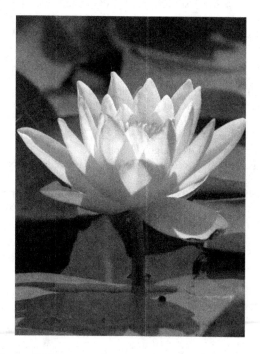

Figure 20.1 Lotus Arising

And by the way, Marquis and I did graduate from Lesley University with our PhD in 2019. My dissertation was entitled: *An Autoethnographic Inquiry of Identity Transformation and Posttraumatic Growth Following Traumatic Brain Injury and PTSD.*

References

Aberjhani, J. (2010). *The river of winged dreams*. Savannah, GA: Black Skylark Singing.

Bunuel, L. (2013). My last sigh: the autobiography of Luis Bunuel. NY: Vintage Books.

Chang, H. (2008). *Autoethnography as method*. Walnut Creek, CA: Left Coast Press.

Genetti, D. (1992). *They forgot I had feelings though I could not feel*. New York, NY: Carlson Press.

Genetti, D. (2023). Identity transformation and posttraumatic growth following traumatic brain injury and posttraumatic stress disorder. New York, NY and Abingdon, OX: Routledge.

Hagen, C., Malkmus, D., Durham, P. (1972). *Levels of cognitive functioning*. Downey, CA: Rancho Los Amigos Hospital.

Kubler-Ross, E. (1997). *On death and dying*. Classic edition. New York City: Scribner Classics.

Maslow, A. (1954). *Motivation and personality*. New York: Harper.

Osborn, C. (1998). *Over my head: A doctor's own story of head injury from the inside looking out*. Kansas City: MO.

Index

abilities, faith (loss) 157
abstinence, maintenance 22
abstract reasoning abilities,
  decrease 155
abuse, power/control
  (involvement) 18
abyss, experience 54
academics, increase 19–23
academic writing, rigor 122
acceptance 155; changes 30
accommodation process,
  occurrence 158
acquired brain injuries 90
activities of daily living (ADLs):
  assistance 46, 67; impairments 44,
  122; strategies, establishment 98
activity (performing), assistance
  (requirement) 45
Act Relative to Cognitive
  Rehabilitation 184–185
acupuncture, usage 125
acute sensations 49
adults with physical disabilities,
  training (providing) 17
agitation 49; ease 71; problem,
  absence 32; reduction 149
AIM Headquarters, membership 16
alternating attention (switching
  attention) 60
alternative solution, usage 41
Alzheimer's Disease 177
ambivalence 157–160
Americans with Disabilities Act (ADA)
  15, 173, 195; compliance 18
analysis 115–119

anecdote, usage 117
anger 71, 141; feeling 118, 119;
  outbursts/surge 70, 110, 133, 141,
  150; problems 68; reckoning 140
anterograde amnesia 28
anxiety 130–131; capacity, reduction
  130; creation 143; plague 178;
  presence 34, 68
Anxiety (Genetti) 131
aphasia 34
appointments, making (difficulty) 76
appreciation: absence 151;
  renewal 179
Aricept (medication), usage 177
arm, muscle sprain 37–38
articulation, need 91
assimilation process, occurrence 158
assistance, requirement 45
assistive strategies, usage 177
assistive technology: Sanders
  reference 97–98; tools, usage 60
assistive technology therapy (AT) 99;
  attending 88–89
assumptions: perception 63–64;
  shattering 151–152
Atech, usage 122–123
attention 60–61; ability, increase
  182; alternating attention
  (switching attention) 60; breaks
  177; capacity, decrease 122;
  complexity 61; difficulty 34,
  38, 39; divided attention 60;
  improvement 149; inability 38;
  increase 45; selective attention 32,
  60, 121; shift 41; span, shortness

33; sustained/focused attention
60; vigilant attention 60
attentional function, impairment 121
attentionally based memory
   impairment, severity 122
attitudes, perception 63–64
auditory information details,
   retention (difficulty) 38
autoethnography 178
autonomy (loss), physical limitation
   (impact) 126
avoidance 68
awakening revelations 49–50
awareness: absence 48; expansion
   52–53; impact 45; impact, increase
   170; increase 86–87, 108

balance, loss 34
bargaining phase 119
behavior: control 67, 124;
   expression 69
behavioral disorganization 122
behavioral issues, concern 169
behavioral skills, relearning 6
benefit finding 171
bill paying: assistance 42; difficulty
   39, 125
"Biological Bases of Behavior"
   research paper 91
body: aches 82; loss 9; transfer,
   difficulty 75–76
booming, experience 49
boom (sound), trigger 133
borderline intelligence 123
brain: capacity, exhaustion 59–60;
   cells, connections (tearing/
   shearing) 37; damage 28, 55, 98;
   emptiness 57–58; energy, diversion
   53; energy, usage 50–51, 53;
   exhaustion 178; fog 48–50, 76;
   functions, coordination (problem)
   41; high-functioning brain injury,
   consideration 43; primary damage
   37; shutdown 48, 51–52, 62;
   strategies, pacing/following 178;
   stretching 179; tissues, bruising/
   swelling 37
brain injury 37, 108, 115, 163, 167;
   dependence 76; impact 42,
   172–173; profile 124; risks

172–173; services 184; workbook,
   usage 178
Brain Injury Association of
   Massachusetts (BIA-MA) 90, 172;
   ambassadorship 183
Brain Injury Checklist, usage 68
breakdown 145; relational
   breakdown 2
break-through events 99–100
breathing: problems 143;
   requirement 99
broken pathways 55
buried alive, feeling 143
business: running, inability 11; skills,
   usage 15
Byers, Julia 161

calculations, difficulties 34, 67
Cambridge Center for Adult
   Education writing course 182
cancer, death 126
car accident dreams 134
car crash: first car crash (1986)
   1, 119; first car crash
   (1986), occurrence/effects
   8–13; occurrence, location
   131–133; re-experiencing
   134; re-experiencing, trigger
   123; second car crash (2007),
   diagnosis/symptoms 27; second
   car crash (2007), occurrence
   27–28
caretaker parental relationship 77
cataclysmic fear 130–131
catastrophic loss 124
categorization worksheet, review
   38–39
censoring 53
centrality, level 156
cervical sprain, treatment 33
change: effort, requirement 110;
   factors, experience 170;
   retraining 110
chronic fatigue 47–48
church bulletin, meditative
   message 159
close head injury, executive function
   deficits 37
clothes: preference, absence 124;
   selection, struggle 39

cognition: capacity, reduction 130; language, interaction 56
cognitive abilities, usage 6
cognitive appraisals (thinking), constructs 156
cognitive capabilities, improvement 169–170
cognitive deficit 63
cognitive disabilities: impact 55–56; invisibility 73, 167
cognitive efficiency, reduction 122
cognitive fatigue 121
cognitive flexibility, impairment 121
cognitive functioning: diminishment 124; levels 30–31
cognitive function, level (recovery) 126
cognitive ideas, integration (attempt) 60
cognitive impairments, severity 121, 124
cognitive linguistic deficit 37
cognitive processing 156
cognitive recommendations 122–123
cognitive rehabilitation bill, testimony 187
cognitive skills 56; metaphor 41; relearning 6
cognitive therapy techniques 37
cohesive ties, weakness 187–188
collaborative relationship 121
collective identity, disability culture (creation) 119
color, rediscovery 100
Committed to a Living Death (Genetti) 130
communication: breakdown 56; deficits 167–168; difficulty 32–33, 70, 83; hallmarks 55; inability, impact 83; language, relationship 56–57; litany, communication 112; miscommunication 57–59; motor function, relationship 63; sensory function, relationship 62; skills, expansion 59–60; skills, loss 2
communities, marginalization 73
Community Access Monitor for Massachusetts, state certification 17
community integration 172–174, 182–183

compassion, difficulties 34
compensatory skills, learning 178
compensatory strategies 163; learning/relearning 88–89
comprehension: ability, loss 54; difficulty 39
concave feeling 64
concentration: absence 89; defining 60; difficulty 38, 39, 54, 68
concurrent mental health issues 120
concussion: diagnosis 32; signs 28–29
confidence: change 171; usage, requirement 119
confusion 29, 45, 49, 108, 145; cause 58; feeling 38; occurrence 37; recognition 32
Connecting Body, Mind and Spirituality (PhD pilot research presentation) 23
consciousness, loss 37, 121
control: absence 64; behavior, control 67; locus, increase 165; loss 86, 143–144; neurological impairment 69
conversations: execution, difficulty 76; futility 84; hearing 49; shortness 143–144; verbal conversation, concentration (absence) 89
co-occurring disorders 141
cooking, supervision (requirement) 121
coping: differences 108; mechanism 45; range 170
coping skills: absence 64; occupational therapy training 145–146; practice 22
cortisone injections, impact 125
counseling responsibilities/passion, increase 19
courage, requirement 119
coworker discrimination 7
creativity, loss 76
cross-disabilities 119
Cry Baby (Joplin) 140
cryptic notes, writing 72, 165

daily functioning: attempt 135; consequences 69

daily living: activities of daily living, impairments 122; basics 76; skills, minimal assistance (requirement) 67
daily newspaper, reading (impossibility) 76
dark glasses, wearing 49
darkness, presence 145
dark place, existence 143
dark shroud, complaint form 49
data analysis, rigors 122
day-end value, absence 86
day planners, usage 163
decision making: capacity, decrease 44; difficulty 44
deep breathing, usage 146
déjà vu, feeling 108
dependence, feeling 123
depression 129–130, 140; deepening 129; depth 143; deterioration 120; feelings 70–71, 147, 167–168; impact 113, 129; journal, usage 70; observation 34, 155; occurrence 118; plague 178; profoundness 126; re-experiencing 122; signs 89; symptoms, struggle 68, 122; thickening 72; worsening 118
depressive feelings, growth 64
despair 141, 142; consumption 145
desperation, feeling 126
detail, identification (trouble) 41
devastation 119
diagnosis 27; changes 30; clinical note 37
difficulties: anticipation, ability 41; handling, inability 171
dignity, occurrence (absence) 151
direction, external input (dependence) 45
disability: advocacy 13–19; core values 196; cultural movement 196; culture 187, 194–197; expense 151
disappointments 64
discrimination 7
disorientation, recognition 32
dissertation, completion 174; determination 43, 118, 178–179
distractibility 68, 121
divided attention 60
dizziness 49; continuation 32

doctoral dissertation (completion), function level (requirement) 126
Doctoral Study Plan (DSP), writing (requirement) 23
domestic violence 8, 13–19
double vision 49, 71
Dragon Dictate, usage 99
Dragon Naturally Speaking (dictation program) 89, 97, 180
dread, feelings 71
dreams 134–139; car accident dreams 134
Dreams (Genetti) 135–136
dressing, execution 45
driving, reactions 133
dying, thoughts 9
dysarthric speech, recognition 32
dysfunction, accrual 15
dyspraxia paresis/plegia 34

eating, execution 45
e-mail, writing (difficulty) 125
EMDR, seeking 118, 123–124
emotional baggage, absence 147
emotional explosion 127
emotional growth 150, 171
emotional ideas, integration (attempt) 60
emotional issues: concern 169; observation 155
emotionality 67, 124, 140; neurological impairment 68–69
emotional stronghold, reduction 116
emotional support 168; loss 77
emotions: articulation 113–114; control, problems 55; unawareness 110
empathy, difficulties 34
employment, difficulty 73
energy: absence 64; low level 76; output, exertion 84; pent up energy, feeling 141; requirement 119
enthusiasm, decrease 89
epiphany 156
Ethel Louise Armstrong Foundation for Leadership in the Disability Community, ELA Scholar award 23
events: external events, victimization 151–152; memory loss 28;

reliving, trauma 123; traumatic
events 126
everyday life, problems 41
executive function: deficits 37; skills,
loss/usage 41
executive functioning: components
56; tasks, variability 121
executive skills: metaphor 41;
utilization 41
exhaustion 54, 119; brain,
exhaustion 178; continuation 64;
display 125
existence, contemplation 152
expectations, structures (change) 133
expressive gestures, usage 56
expressive-receptive abilities,
problems 56
external events, victimization 151–152

facial expressions, usage 54
facial gestures, usage 56
failure 64; fear 167
faith, rediscovery 6
familial relationships, strains 78–82
family: counseling, providing 21;
members, closeness (increase)
179; split 13; violence, survivors
(responses) 20–21
Family (Genetti) 79–80
fate, acceptance 118–119
father, condition (problems)
192–193
fatigue 58, 111, 172; chronic fatigue
47–48; cognitive fatigue 121;
difficulty 39, 68; focus 101; instant
fatigue 51–52; inundation 54;
management 180; occurrence 38,
42, 53–54; physical fatigue 47;
post exertional fatigue 50–53;
rapid fatigue 122; repetition 61;
signs 89; testing, cessation 121
fear 147, 150; cataclysmic fear
130–131; feelings 71, 133;
presence 77
Fear (Genetti) 138–139
feedback 92, 183, 188
feelings: hatred 141; log, usage 60;
negative feelings, management 22
filtering 53
financial strains, decrease 77

first car crash (1986) 1, 119;
occurrence/effects 8–13
flashbacks 106, 131–134, 146;
continuation 148; control, absence
135; impact 127; intrusion 89;
invasion 32, 70; notes *132*;
suffering 12
focal neurological deficit 34
focus, loss 89
fog 71, 107, 160; roll 49
food, preference (absence) 124
footpath, discovery 88
forgetfulness 83
forward-thinking, ability
(challenge) 103
fragmented responses 31–32
fragments, writing 96
free-writing 49–50
frenzy, feeling 141
fresh air, love 141
friends, assistance 82–83
friendships, creation 179
frontal lobe: headache 58;
impact 37
frustration 53, 110; catching
119; tolerance, low level
(observation) 155
full thoughts, writing (goal) 91
functional abilities, decline 89
functional status, decrease 121

Gere, Susan 161
gestures, usage 56
goal-directed patient, observations 177
goals, defining 116
God: accompaniment 160; anger 71,
158; connectedness 159; faith,
loss 157; fate 158; impact, reasons
150; presence 10
"going-out-the-door list" 98
grace, occurrence (absence) 151
grasping words, usage 95
gratitude list, creation 179
Greater Boston Chamber of
Commerce, membership 7
grief 9; stages 45, 71–72, 155;
writing 188–192
grocery shopping, assistance 40
growth: anticipation 171–172;
discovery 177

haiku, creation 73
handicapped people: treatment 10; world, inaccessibility 14–15
hand, pain 140
handwriting tasks, residual motor impairments (impact) 63
happiness: disappearance 119; feeling, absence 151
head: disorganization 82; emptiness 48; holding, difficulty 54; inflammation, treatment 32; injuries, continuation 67; spasms, assessment 33
headaches 28, 49, 108; frontal lobe headache 58; occurrence, ease 38; severity 76
Head Trauma Program of the Rusk Institute of Rehabilitation Medicine (HTP) 104; attendees, self (loss) 113; exercises 117–118; lecture, writing (Osborn) 115; Osborn attendance 106; Osborn graduation 111; survivor group, recovery 115
healing process, learning 6
healing rose garden 109f
hearing, changes 34
heart, pounding 134, 144
Heller, Caroline 161
helplessness 167; feeling 123, 151
Hierarchy of Basic Needs (Maslow) 93
higher-level processing problems, difficulty 38
high-functioning brain injury, consideration 43
high-level language organization, difficulty 122
HITS Fund, collections 184
hobbies, development 147
holistic presentation, retention (inability) 38
home: disorganization 125; imprisonment 11; minimal function, maintenance 42; quietude 53–54
hope: loss 118; positive emotion 157; presence 118; strengthening 149
hopelessness, feeling 126
horror, feeling 86

household: activities, performing (safety) 121; chaos 42
house, ramp (installation) 16
humiliation 167
humor, sense (loss) 76
hyperarousal 68
hyper-vigilance 133

identity: loss 73, 116; transformation 30
I Did Not Go (Genetti) 149
impairments: acknowledgment 155; groups 69; hiding 117
impatient rehabilitation 145
imprisonment 13–19
incomplete thoughts, writing 96
independence levels, diversity 166
independent function, impossibility 125
independent living skills, loss 2
individual counseling, providing 21
information: accumulation, absence 33; acquisition/retrieval, ability (reduction) 122; efficiency, deficit 52; filtering, energy (need) 53; noise/static, comparison 164–165; synthesis/analysis, functional ability (loss) 42
information processing 95; change 42; learning 43; problems/deficit 30, 52
injury: debilitation 125; impairments 101; permanence 150
injury-related issues 192
in-patient therapies 145–148
insight, discovery 177
insomnia 47–48
instant fatigue 51–52
instinctive motivations, reliance 160
integrated psychotherapy 2
intellect 67; neurological impairment 68–69
intellectual impairments 69
intellectual responsibilities, performing 62
interests, development 147
interference: contribution 57; occurrence 133
interpersonal difficulties 68

interpersonal relationships: changes 67, 74; difficulties 73
interpersonal skills, relearning 6
interpretation 115–119
intrusive thoughts, management 22
iPad magnifier, usage 165
IQ, testing 123
irritability: ease 71; observation 155; presence 68
I Shine (Genetti) 192
isolation, feeling 86

JAWS (speech program) 98
job, execution (impossibility) 117
joint body aches 54
Joplin, Janis 140
judgment, difficulty 34

Keller, Helen 5
Keverian, George 185
knowledge: scrambling 44; thirst 7

language: cognition, interaction 56; communication, relationship 56–57; expression, difficulty 34; high-level language organization, difficulty 122; impairments 121–122; problems, difficulty 38
laundry, sorting (inability) 142
learning: difficulty 45; rediscovery 6; tools, collection 37
left arm, usage 29, 126
legs, paralysis 29
Lesley University: BS/MA program, acceptance 20; Doctoral Teaching Fellowship, receipt 23; PhD program 23
lethargy, occurrence 32
Licensed Mental Health Counselor (LMHC), attainment 20, 172–173
life: blur 151; change 2, 75, 119; change, brain injury (impact) 42; confusion 145; control, absence 64; course, change 150; demands, adjustment (assistance) 169; direction 144; gift, blessing 159; God, accompaniment 160; loss 6; meaning, finding 170; nature, understanding 159; new life 118–119; patterned routines 101;

quality, absence 142; satisfaction, growth 178; theme 8; traumatic events 126; verb, usage 143; worth, rebuilding (impact) 119
Life-changing Crash (Genetti) 190–191
life coach: discovery 90–94; impact 88
lifestyle, relearning 102–103
light, sensitivity 49
limbs: ability/use, loss 126; left arm, usage 29, 126; physical pain 64
limitations: acceptance 115–116; understanding 116
list making, difficulty 124
litany, communication 112
Living stories (workshop) 183
loneliness, articulation (difficulty) 83
long-range thought 107

mail, sorting: assistance 42; struggle 39
main idea, identification (difficulty) 44
main sentences, deciphering 91
Major Depressive Disorder (MDD) 91, 145; defining 115; depression, worsening 118
Massachusetts Clearinghouse of Mutual Self Help Groups, membership 16
Massachusetts Coalition for Citizens with Disabilities, membership 16
Massachusetts Commission for the Blind (MCB), work 17
Massachusetts Eye and Ear Infirmary (MEEI), testing/confirmation 17
Massachusetts Rehabilitation Commission (MRC) 94; Protective Services Unit 18, 20
material, learning organization 97
maximalist thinking 114
me: belief, loss 125; loss 6, 118, 125; nonacceptance 64
meaning: recognition 180–181; sense 160; structures, change 133
meaning, finding: attainment 170; desire 150
medications: setup 81; side effect 145; usage 40

medicine, changes 115
memory 59–60; absence 56; capacity, increase 177; capacity, reduction 130, 185–186; compensatory strategies 60; deficits 167–168; difficulty 32–34, 38, 46, 122–123; difficulty, recognition 32; fade 47; impairment 32; improvement 149; increase 45; integration 148; letting go 110; log, usage 60; loss 28, 37, 169; notebook, usage 60; photographic memory, loss 43; placeholder, usage 149; problems 82; reduction 122; repair 112; short-term memory, impairment 124; tribulations, anxiety 130; troubles 68; working memory, problems 96, 149
mental clipboard, problems 30, 57–58
mental health issues 120
mental impairment, treatment 86
mentor, discovery 90–94
Merrimack Valley Coalition of Disabled Advocates, board membership 17
Miceli, James 185
mild traumatic brain injury (mTBI) 34, 121
milieu support, providing 21
mind: absence 107; awakening 160; blankness 34
mirror image feelings 113–114
miscommunication 57–59; social miscommunication, occurrence 59
misery, escape 141
mobility impairment 167
mood: changes 137; disorders 69–70
morals, rethinking 160
morning clarity, absence 50
mortality: facing 164; sense 167
motor function, communication (relationship) 63
motor systems 122
multiple tasks, juggling (difficulty) 42
multi-step problems, solving (difficulties) 67
multitasking, loss 99
muscle: aches 51–52, 54; sprain 37–38

muscular flexibility, physical stretches (usage) 37
mutuality 92

Namenda (medication), usage 177
nausea 134; continuation 32
neck: inflammation, treatment 32; injuries, continuation 67; injury 125; spasms, assessment 33; sprain 29, 37–38
negative energy, release 140–141
negative feelings, management 22
negative self-perception, permanence 42
nerve impingements 125–126
neurological impairments, brain injury (impact) 68–69
neurological problems 69
neuropsychological evaluation 120–123
neuropsychological testing 126
new life 118–119
Newman, Daniel 161
new normal, finding 155
nightmares 70, 135; control, absence 135; notes *132*; suffering 12
Nighttime Fright (Genetti) 136–137
noise 54, 58; blending 49; impact 133
Northeast Independent Living Program (NILP): in-service meetings 18; part-time work 16–17
note-taking 95–96; devices, usage 163; strategies (Sanders) 102–103
note, writing (attempt) 58
nothingness fog 49
novel reasoning ability, intactness 121

occupational therapy (OT) 147; attendance 88; training 145
old self: loss 31–35, 64; memories, fading 116
one-sentence prediction/question 102
one-step direction, limitations 76
ongoing pain, effects 122
Open Space and Recreation Commission, membership 173
optimism: gaining 165; increase 165
organic problem, brain injury (impact) 110

Osborn, Claudia 102, 104, 111, 181; comparison 112; depression, impact 113; journal quote 112; recovery paradigm 115; transparency 114; turning point 118; work 115
others: anger 71; dependency 76
outbursts, anger 110
outpatient therapy rehabilitation, usage 31
Over My Head (Osborn) 84, 102, 103, 115; commonalities 106–111; contrasts/comparison 103–107; therapy 94
overstimulation 76, 143
overwhelmedness 58; vacillation 49

pacing 140
pain, knowledge 12
palpitations, experience 134
panel speaker 162–166; presentation 162; rehearsal 164–165
panic 42–43
paralysis 9
paraplegia 8
passageways, opening 177
patience, absence 86
patient: improvement 44; safety, supervision (requirement) 67
pectoral muscles: injuries, continuation 67; injury 125; spasms 33, 125–126
pentup energy, feeling 141
perfectionism 107
peripheral visual fields, loss 49
permanent, term (usage) 113
perseveration, evidence 121
personal activities of daily living, assistance (requirement) 46
personal assistant (PA), interaction 74
personality: changes/alterations 34, 69; factors 171–172; traits/limitations 77
personal meaning, sense (growth) 178
personal vulnerability, exposure 145
persona, schema (loss) 171
philosophy, changes 30
phone calling, difficulty 61, 76
photographic memory, loss 30, 43
photophobia 68

phrases, listening/speaking 99
physical access, liberation (comparison) 16
physical disability, permanence 14
physical fatigue 47
physical limitations, feeling 75
physical mobility, absence 75
physical needs, self-care (inability) 46
physical pain 64
physical therapy (PT): continuation 162; exercises 92; impact 146; usage 33
physical writing, difficulty 123
physiological impairments 69–70
pictures, finding (difficulty) 38–39
plan, execution (difficulty) 44
plants, care/ability (loss) 76
pleasurable, acceptance 118
pleasure, feeling 118
poetic journey 181
positivity, absence 63
post-acute care cognitive rehabilitation, coverage (absence) 31
post-concussion syndrome (PCS): diagnosis 32, 34; treatment 33
post exertional fatigue 50–53
post-it notes, reading 141
post-traumatic brain injury (post-TBI) 31–35; interpersonal relationships, changes 67
post-traumatic growth (PTG) 5, 63, 74, 178; causes 171; factors 160, 181; fostering 165–166; impact 172; phenomenon 193; report 151; result 157; theory 6
post-traumatic stress 171
post-traumatic stress disorder (PTSD) 1, 150; co-morbidity 129; co-occurrence 5; defining 115; episodes 127; gender/culture 167–168; multiple traumas, relationship 122; outlook, gloom 12; reactions 122; re-experiencing 122; symptomatology 118; treatment 148
powerlessness 167; feeling 127
power, loss 86
power wheelchair, usage 33, 75–76
Predict-Read-Prove method 102
pre-primers, continuation 43

pride, loss 84–85
priorities, decision making
    (difficulties) 44
prioritization, inability 124
problems: recognition, involvement
    41; solving 41
problem-solving difficulties 68
processing, learning 43
procrastination, effect 125
psychological consequences 69–71
psychotherapy, continuation 123–128
PTGI assessment tool 193
purpose: return 161; sense,
    development 178

quadriplegia, possibility 28
quietness/stillness, existence 179

rage: impact 142; outpouring
    110, 127
Rancho Los Amigos Recovery Scale
    (RLAS) 45, 67, 155, 169
Rancho Los Amigos Recovery Scale
    of Cognitive Functioning 31–32
rapid fatigue 122
rational judgments, difficulties 67
Ray of Hope, A (Genetti) 80–81
reading: cessation 96; comprehension,
    difficulty 91; deficits 37; difficulty
    36–37, 49; learning 95; post-it
    notes, reading 141
reasoning: abstract reasoning
    abilities, decrease 155; difficulty
    34; novel reasoning ability,
    intactness 121; repair 112
reciprocal lobe, impact 37
recognition: flaws/complexity
    97; tasks, performance
    (problems) 122
recording file, transcription 99
recovery 101, 197; completion,
    outpatient therapy rehabilitation
    (usage) 31; lifelong learning 31;
    paradigm 115; prognosis 126;
    road 112; story, structure 30–31;
    work 151
refocus, time (requirement) 54
rehabilitation: goal 43; life coach,
    impact 88; path 148–149;
    program 114

re-identification 67–71, 115–119;
    changes 30; initiation 112
relational breakdown 2
relationships 73; changes 30;
    changes, confirmation 77;
    closeness 74–76, 81; decrease
    86; development 92; impact
    83–84; increase 179; interference,
    occurrence 133; problems 22;
    renewal 120; reversal 75; suffering
    53–54
relaxation 143
relearning 116
religious faith, affirmation 179
residual motor impairments,
    impact 63
resilience: absence 64; gaining 170
restlessness, occurrence 32, 70
restorative rest, demand 52–53
rest periods: focus 101; importance
    52–53
right arm, pain 134
right shoulder: orthopedic/
    neurological infractions 9; sprain,
    treatment 33; usage, absence 108
rotator cuff pain 125, 134
rotator cuff tear 28, 108, 162;
    treatment 33
role changes 77
routine changes, disorientation
    69–70
rubber balls, throwing (therapy)
    70, 140
rudimentary motor control
    (tasks), stimulus bound behavior
    (evidence) 121
rumination 157–160; loop,
    observation 157
ruminative brooding, actions 150,
    156–157, 159

Sadness and Grief I Can't Handle
    (Genetti) 12–13
sadness, feelings 167–168
safety: goal 22; supervision,
    requirement 67
Sanders, R. Richard 44, 49, 57–62,
    90–91; assistive technology
    reference 97–98; cognitive work
    158; conversations 170; graduate

students 163; guidance 93–94;
interaction 99; mentorship 92;
note-taking template 102–103;
progress note 148–149; Rick list,
usage 165; Speech-Language
Pathology Daily Note 187;
summary reports 71
screaming 91, 140, 142
second car crash (2007): diagnosis/
symptoms 27; occurrence 27–28
Seeking Safety (group protocol) 22
selective attention 60; impairment
32, 121
self: anger 71; fragmentation/
integration 30; journey, stages
30; loss 55, 113, 118, 181; old
self, loss 31–35, 64; old self,
memories (fading) 116; shell
(comparison) 38, 117; spiritual
self, reorganization 170
self-actualization 93
self-assuredness 170
self-awareness: gaining 169; goal 89;
relearning 41
self-care activities, patient
performance 67
self-concept, change 171
self-discovery, initiation 101
self-esteem, increase 165
self-evaluative journal entry 64
self-expression, inability 83
self-help, knowledge (absence) 143
self-identification, TBI (impact) 151
self-monitoring, difficulty 40–41, 155
self-observational data, capture/
collection 1
self-observations 146
self-perception, changes 30, 31–35, 57
self-pity, wallowing 64
self-reliance, sense (loss) 171
self-representation, problems 87
self-respect 93
self-understanding/self-respect,
increase 22
self-worth 93
senses, overload 54
sensory acuteness 49
sensory changes 38
sensory function, communication
(relationship) 62

sentences: completion, attempt
86; dissection, learning 59;
main sentences, deciphering
91; proofreading 96; structure
95–96; supporting sentences,
deciphering 91; understanding,
difficulty 59; whole sentences,
writing 96
sentences, writing 96; ability, goal
91; learning 107
sequelae, co-occurrence 118
service dog (Othello) 91; love/
assistance, gratefulness 179;
presence 33, 103–104
shadows, haunting 118
shame 59; feelings 133
short-term memory, impairment
38, 124
shoulder: injuries, continuation 67;
muscle sprain 37–38; pain 125;
right shoulder, usage (absence) 108;
spasms, assessment 33; sprain 29
siblings, protection 13
sight, changes 34
situations, control (need) 41–42
skill-oriented tasks, performing 62
skills, improvement (learning) 178
sleep: craving 47–48, 84; flashbacks,
invasion 70; maintenance,
problems 122
sleep apnea 70, 122
social actions 183–186
social context 119
social cues, interpretation
(difficulty) 55
social desolation, creation 83
social devaluation 86
social interaction 74
social miscommunication,
occurrence 59
social opportunities, decrease 77
social outreach, impact 167
social supports: increase 179;
limitation 2
solved problem, response pattern
(shift) 41
sorrow, intensity 38
soul-searching 119, 159
sounds: amplification 32, 49, 62;
hearing 49

Spaulding Rehabilitation Hospital, therapies 89, 91, 94
speech: continuation 37; deceleration 85–86; difficulty 37; experience 164; slow rate 84; understanding 45
speech impediment 49; assistance 37
speech-language: emphasis 164; training 99
speech-language-cognitive therapy (ST) 88, 92, 162
speech-language pathology clinical specialist, strategies 98
Speech-Language Pathology Daily Note (Sanders) 187
speech-language therapy 36; continuation 41
speech therapy 127–128; sessions, continuation 57
spinal cord, severing 9
spine injury, absence 29
spirit: access 158–159; crushing 64; liberation 158
Spirit of Tranquility, The (Genetti) 109–110
spiritual crisis 155
spiritual decline 149–151
spiritual enlightenment 159
spiritual growth 150
spirituality, meaningfulness/ strengthening 170
spiritual matters, understanding 160
spiritual self, reorganization 170
spiritual values, affirmation 179
stamina, low level 76
standby assistance: request 169; requirement 155
startle response, sensitization 133
Statewide Advisory Council for Protective Services, MRC initiation (charter membership) 18
status, disorganization 124
stepping stones, unearthing 95
stigma 85–86
stimulation, tolerance 58
stimulus bound behavior, evidence 121
story, transcendence 161
strengths, vision (accuracy) 41
stress: capacity, reduction 130; negative outcomes 171
stress-related growth 171

stuttering 30, 32, 81, 84
Sub-Humans, The (Genetti) 10–11, 85
subject, condensation 162–163
subject-verb-object 96
substance abuse problems, treatment 21
successful, term (redefining) 116–117
suffering 143; aftermath 130; articulation 113–114
suffering groups 69
suicidal feelings 142, 149
suicidal ideation 12, 118, 140, 143
suicidality 12
suicide, completion (likeliness) 129
summarization, inability 40–41
summary, writing (ability) 97
support group 105–106, 166–167
supporting sentences, deciphering 91
Supreme Insidious Ache, A (Genetti) 137–138
surface clutter, organization (struggle) 39
survivors, recovery 86
sustained attention: impairment 121; problem 37
sustained/focused attention 60
sweating 134
symptomatology 112, 118

Taken, The (Genetti) 188–190
talking, problems 29–30
tangentiality, evidence 124
tasks: accomplishment, energy requirement 42; concentration, difficulty 61; coping, inability 123; handling 177; skill-oriented tasks, performing 62
taste, changes 34
teeth brushing, execution 45
temples, pulsation 29
therapy: appointments/homework/ practices 46; exercises 327; work 44
They Forgot I Had Feelings Though I Could Not Feel (Genetti) 12, 73, 78–79
thinking: disabilities, impact 55–56; forward-thinking, ability (challenge) 103; maximalist thinking 114; repair 112; tiredness 53; trouble 76

thoughts: articulation 113–114; assembly, inability 29–30; bad thoughts 86; deciphering, inability 33; exhaustion 50; explanation 96; flood 110; full thoughts, writing (goal) 91; incomplete thoughts, writing 96; intrusive thoughts, management 22; long-range thought 107; loss 149; manipulation, problems 59–60; multiplicity, holding (ability) 178; organization, inability 125; outpouring 58; regaining, goal 63; shifting patterns, relearning 41

throat, inflammation (treatment) 32

time: blur 36; loss 48–49, 84; obliviousness 45

timed thought generation, impairment 121

tiredness 99–100, 143

tissues, bruising/swelling 37

to-do lists, usage 60

tolerance, absence 144

train of thought, loss 149

tranquility 109

transcendence 161

transportation numbers/names, usage 60

trauma: experiences, encapsulation 188; exposure 158; memories, integration 148; negative outcomes 171; patterns, repetition/reoccurrence 14; re-experiencing 122; survivors, psychological experiences (experience) 156; therapy 20; working 150

traumata, understanding 180–181

trauma-therapist self, healing 114

Traumatic Brain Injury (TBI): challenges/catastrophe 2; co-morbidity 129; context, setting 5; defining 115; disability culture 104; episodes 127; feeling 116; gender/culture 167–168; mild traumatic brain injury (mTBI) 34, 121; negative connotation/stigma, change 2; ramifications, awareness 155; recovery 1–2; rehabilitation 172; result, impact 126; sub-culture 104–105

Traumatic Brain Injury (TBI) survivors: depletion, feeling 73; meeting/hearing 164–165

traumatic closed brain injury 37

traumatic losses, grief 155–156

traumatic stress disorder, symptoms 32

trigger point injections, usage 125

trust 92; ability, loss 125

turning point 118

typographic errors (typos), multiplicity 108

ulna nerve, orthopedic/neurological infractions 9

unconscious motivations, reliance 160

understanding skills, expansion 59–60

unresolved issues, recycling 125

unsteadiness 100

upbeat person, decrease 89

upper back, orthopedic/neurological infractions 9

Upside-Down Turtle, The (Genetti) 101–102

value, discovery 177

Venn Diagram *103*

verbal conversation, concentration (absence) 89

verbal expression, difficulty 122

verbal fluency, reduction 122

verbalization, cues (requirement) 149

verbal responses, hesitation 89

verbosity, mildness 149

vibrancy, decrease 89

victimization, admission (refusal) 14

vigilant attention 60

violation, feelings 133

visceral connections 110

visible expressions, display 89

vision: blurriness 32, 71; change 34, 49; double vision 49, 71

visual constructional ability, impairment 122

visual guided imageries 146

visual impairment 167

visual scanning 62

voice: physical stretches, usage 37;
  silence 9
vomiting 28
vulnerability (feeling): hatred 171;
  personal vulnerability, exposure
  145; physical limitation,
  impact 126

wallowing, avoidance 119
weakness 48
weaknesses: vision, accuracy 41
weariness 64
wheelchair: battery, cessation 142;
  knowledge 21–22; lift, problem
  167; power wheelchair, usage 33,
  75–76; scrutiny 19; transfers 81;
  usage/demonstration 14–15, 85
Wheelchair-bound (Genetti) 11
Wheelchair Grievances (Genetti) 9
wheelchair transfer assistance 76
Wheelman, The (Genetti)
  19–20, 131
whiplash, diagnosis 32
whole sentences, writing 96
Wilmington ADA Committee,
  appointment 17
Wilmington Commission on
  Disabilities: chairing 173;
  membership 16
Wilmington Committee for Citizens
  with Disabilities (WCCD) 185;
  membership 16

wisdom: consideration 162;
  development 181–182
withdrawal, requirement 119
womanhood, future issues (fear) 167
Women Embracing Life and Living
  (WELL) project 21
words: finding difficulties/problems
  37, 68, 82–83, 93; grasping
  words, usage 95; pauses 89;
  retrieval deficits 122
work: doctoring 96; ethic, strength
  7, 107; gains, impenetrability
  120–121
working memory, problems 96, 149
worksheets, usage 95
world: physical access, liberation
  (comparison) 16; reconnection 56
Wrath of Death, The (Genetti) 127
writing: clarity, increase 177; desire
  108; difficulty 58; facilitation 122–
  123; fragments, writing 96; free-
  writing 49–50; improvement 187–
  188; inability 140; incomplete
  thoughts, writing 96; learning 95;
  paragraphs, addition (attempt)
  108; physical writing, difficulty
  123; sentences, learning 107;
  sentences, writing ability (goal) 91;
  skills, requirement 63
written language, difficulty 37

zoning out 50, 71, 76

Printed in the United States
by Baker & Taylor Publisher Services